Nursing as Therapy

Nursing as Therapy

Edited by

Richard McMahon

Senior Nurse
Horton General Hospital
Banbury and Lecturer Practitioner, Oxford Polytechnic

and

Alan Pearson

Professor of Nursing and Foundation Dean
Deakin University
Victoria, Australia

CHAPMAN & HALL

London · Glasgow · New York · Tokyo · Melbourne · Madras

Published by Chapman & Hall, 2-6 Boundary Row, London SE1 8HN, UK

Chapman & Hall, 2-6 Boundary Row, London SE1 8HN, UK

Blackie Academic & Professional, Wester Cleddens Road, Bishopbriggs, Glasgow G64 2NZ, UK

Chapman & Hall Inc., One Penn Plaza, 41st Floor, New York, NY10119, USA

Chapman & Hall Japan, Thomson Publishing Japan, Hirakawacho Nemoto Building, 6F, 1-7-11 Hirakawa-cho, Chiyoda-ku, Tokyo 102, Japan

Chapman & Hall Australia, Thomas Nelson Australia, 102 Dodds Street, South Melbourne, Victoria 3205, Australia

Chapman & Hall India, R. Seshadri, 32 Second Main Road, CIT East, Madras 600 035, India

First edition 1991
Reprinted 1992, 1993

© 1991 Richard McMahon and Alan Pearson

Typeset in 10½/12pt Palatino by Mews Photosetting, Beckenham, Kent
Printed in Great Britain by St Edmundsbury Press Ltd, Bury St Edmunds

ISBN 0 412 35440 3

A catalogue record for this book is available from the British Library

Library of Congress Cataloging-in-Publication data available

Contents

Contributors

Steven Ersser, BSc (Hons), RGN Post Graduate Research Student, Institute of Nursing, Oxford/King's College, London.

Jillian MacGuire, BA, PhD, RGH RCN Professor of Nursing Research, University of Wales College of Medicine.

Christine C. McKee, RGN, DN(Cert), PWT, Dip N, Cert Ed RNT Lecturer Practitioner, South West College of Health Studies, Barncoose Hospital, Redruth.

Richard McMahon, MA, Dip N, RGN Senior Nurse, Horton General Hospital, Banbury; also Lecturer Practitioner, Oxford Polytechnic.

Alan Pearson, SRN, ONC, Dip N Ed, DANS, MSc, PhD, Professor of Nursing and Foundation Dean, School of Nursing, Deakin University, Geelong, Victoria, Australia.

Jean Powell, MSc, DNT, RNT, RGN Head of Department of Health Studies, Buckinghamshire College of Higher Education.

Elizabeth Tutton, MSc, BSc (Hons), RGN, PGCEA Principal Lecturer, Buckinghamshire College of Higher Education.

Barbara Vaughan, SRN, RCNT, RNT, DIP N(Lond), DANS, MSc Senior Lecturer in Nursing Studies, University of Wales College of Medicine.

Stephen Wright, RGN, RCNT, Dip N, RNT, DANS, MSc Consultant Nurse, Tameside General Hospital.

Preface

Over the past 20 years, nursing has begun to rediscover some of its basic 'truths' which have become obscured because of the rise in technology and medical knowledge this century. One of these basic 'truths' is the concern of this book – that intelligent, sensitive nursing does make a difference to the consumers of health care. Like most essential truths, this seems almost too obvious to be stated. Nevertheless, many nurses have become increasingly aware of a commonly held view that 'getting better' or staying healthy is largely dependent upon the intervention of or monitoring by medical practitioners and paramedical therapists together with the technology they use and that nurses merely carry out the orders of such workers and keep things in order. An apt analogy, frequently used, is that of the air journey. The point of the journey is to get from A to B and is largely dependent upon the aeroplane (i.e. the technology in health care) and the crew in the cockpit (i.e. the doctor as pilot and the paramedical therapists as co-pilots, navigator and engineer when equated to health care). In this analogy, nurses are seen as analogous to the cabin crew – the flight attendants who make the journey more comfortable and bearable, but who could really be done without in getting from A to B, even though they are nice to have around. Many would argue however, that the analogy is not at all apt. Nursing is not like the work of flight attendants and is not merely something nice to have around. Its impact on the journey is equal to that of the doctor and paramedical therapists; its actions are indeed therapeutic – nursing is yet another form of therapy.

This latter view is held by the writers in this book which has as its central concern the notion that a certain form of nursing has a powerful effect on health and healing. For example, it is important for the modern world to realise that prior to the advent of antibiotics, a sizeable number of people suffering from severe pneumonia recovered from that illness as a result of the interventions of nurses. At that time, there were no other forms of therapy for such patients and nurses provided comfort, nourishment, chest percussion and postural drainage, an environment of care, and numerous interventions to enable the person to engage in essential physical, social and emotional processes to maintain life and overcome the disease by mobilising the body's own natural resources.

This somewhat simple truism that nursing is therapeutic, and nursing's recent rediscovery of it, has led to the rise of the concept of 'therapeutic nursing' or 'nursing as therapy'. As yet, our understandings and explorations of this remain to be developed. In this book, our developing ideas are laid open to the reader for discussion, challenge and further development.

In Chapter 1, the scene is set and the historical development of this emerging concept is outlined. Further chapters focus on specific issues which arise out of this history. The book does not develop a recipe on how to be therapeutic, nor does it clearly delineate what nursing as therapy actually is. To do so would be impossible as well as arrogant and pre-emptive. What it does attempt to do is to offer a number of perspectives which scrutinise the concept and which give pointers to what is therapeutic in nursing, and to future directions which will exploit the therapeutic potential embodied in the process of nursing.

As nursing is still a predominantly female profession, the pronoun she is used throughout to refer to the nurse whilst the pronoun he, to the patient. This is in no way intended to slight many worthy male nurses or female patients!

Richard McMahon
Alan Pearson, Oxfordshire

Foreword

LISBETH HOCKEY

My first reaction to the term 'therapeutic nursing' was negative. At best, I considered it a tautology on the basis that all nursing is, or at least should be, therapeutic. At worst, I perceived it as another example of jargon, by which I mean *unnecessary* technical terminology. The jargon or 'new speak' vogue which seems to have invaded nursing tends to evoke a negative reaction in me and often stops me from thinking further about the term used. It was an invitation to address the first British conference on 'therapeutic nursing' in Oxford in March 1989 which provided the impetus for a serious study of the term and its origin. My preparation for that conference gave me insights for which I am grateful. This foreword is based on the paper delivered on that occasion and I accepted the editors' invitation to contribute to their exciting book with pleasure and an awareness of the honour and privilege afforded to me.

In his classic work on the French revolution, the great historian Eric Hobsbaum said: 'Words are witnesses which often speak louder than documents' (Hobsbaum 1962). He referred to some English words which either made their debut in the English vocabulary or took on new meanings. He felt that the need for new words or new meanings demonstrates the beginnings of a new era, a new trend, a new process. The term 'therapeutic nursing' seems a good example. It is possible, therefore, that the new term heralded a new activity – a new type of nursing. It is equally possible that the activity existed before but, owing to the lack of an appropriate descriptive term, it was not recognised, that it shared a similar fate to the process of nursing or the 'nursing process'.

How one views these possibilities or what one identifies as the activity of therapeutic nursing clearly depends on one's interpretation of it. A definition seems essential before any claim for the practice of therapeutic nursing can be made.

Neither the English dictionaries nor the professional literature shed light on a clear definition. The term 'therapy', 'therapeia' is explained as 'medical treatment' derived from the Greek. The adjective 'therapeutic' is described as meaning 'curative' or 'of the healing art'. The definition of the noun 'therapeutics' is 'branch of medicine concerned with treatment of disease and action of remedial agents in disease or health'. It seems that the intent of those who propound therapeutic nursing is to show that nursing can be used as a remedial agent, that it can be curative or healing.

Therapeutics, as a science, is not specific to nursing; it is an important part of many aspects of health care.

Nursing has been described as the art of applying nursing science, nursing science being a unique mix of other underlying sciences, the uniqueness lying in the mix (Hockey 1979).

It follows that, providing the scientific principles of therapeutics are part of the nursing syllabus, their application to nursing activities will bring them into the nursing arena.

Therapeutic nursing can now be explained as the practice of those nursing activities which have a healing effect or those which result in a movement towards health or wellness. It is important to emphasise that both 'healing' and 'health' must be regarded as multidimensional, and should include physical, emotional, spiritual, mental and environmental considerations. Such a wide interpretation allows therapeutic nursing to be offered as part of terminal care.

Unlike 'therapeutic nursing', the terms 'holistic nursing' and 'holism' appear frequently in the nursing literature of many western countries, including the UK. Both concepts are based on the same all-embracing interpretation of health, which might explain why holistic nursing and therapeutic nursing are often used interchangeably. My view is that holistic nursing, the care of the 'whole person', is a necessary but not a sufficient condition of therapeutic nursing. It is impossible to move a patient or client toward total health if the importance of total health is not acknowledged. It cannot be taken for granted, however, that holistic nursing is, by definition, therapeutic or that it is the only possible healing strategy that can be used. Holistic nursing is a necessary condition because of the inseparable relationships between body, mind, spirit and the environment. Their influences on each other are well known.

If the above explanation of 'therapeutic nursing' is accepted, its use in modern nursing seems defensible. It is a new term expressing a new way of looking at nursing.

The possibility of 'therapeutic nursing' being a tautology on the grounds that all nursing is therapeutic was, after all, dispelled by Florence Nightingale, when she said:

'If a patient is cold, if a patient is feverish, if he is sick after taking food, if he has a bedsore, it is generally the fault, not of the disease, but of the nursing' (Nightingale 1852).

She claimed that poor nursing interrupted nature's process of repairing the body, resulting in pain and other forms of suffering. It follows that there must be a type of nursing which cannot be blamed for such consequences and which, on the contrary, can hasten the patient's restoration to a measure of health or, at least, ameliorate or control undesirable sensations and symptoms. This type of nursing, which moves a patient towards 'health' in its widest sense, is referred to as 'therapeutic'.

It is gratifying that several of the models now offered as conceptual images of nursing make provision for the multidimensional aspects of health. In addition, the model, based on the activities of living, expounded by Roper et al. (1985), incorporates specifically the movement of patients along the axis to health/independence.

Having suggested that 'therapeutic nursing' is a viable concept, it remains to identify its content. It is also necessary to provide evidence of the therapeutic value claimed. Conventional and innovative practices must be submitted to scientific scrutiny if they are to be taken seriously as contributing to healing or health. Altschul's (1972) work on patient–nurse interactions was seminal in this respect. She rightly questioned the therapeutic value of nurse–patient relationships in the field of psychiatric nursing. The concept of 'therapeutic relationship' can clearly be applied to all branches of nursing. It is impossible to nurse a patient without some sort of relationship with him or her, but it can be healing or harmful. Therefore, a calculated relationship purporting to have a healing effect is a fundamental form of therapeutic nursing, providing the purpose is achieved and demonstrated. Touch is another fundamental area of nursing and its therapeutic potential is receiving increasing attention (Wolanin and Phillips 1981, Redfern and Le May 1986). Thus, therapeutic relationships and therapeutic touch are examples of a specified purpose of conventional direct nursing. Increasingly, however, new complementary therapies are referred to in the context of therapeutic nursing and their range is multiplying at a phenomenal rate. They include activities such as aromatherapy, meditation, imagery, acupuncture, reflexology, applied kinesiology, yoga, biofeedback, Alexander techniques, macrobiotic diet, hypnosis, irridology and others (Rankin-Box 1988).

Whether these procedures constitute nursing or not is an important, but as yet unanswered, question. It seems to me that both stances can be defended, depending on the total situation. If the complementary therapies are carried out as part of an enlarged repertoire of a nurse, they are indisputably nursing; the only proviso must be that they have been taught within the context of nursing science including the art of their appropriate application. If they are administered independent from nursing, not as part of the nursing care plan, they are probably not nursing. This position does not imply that nurses have to give all the new therapies themselves in order for them to be part of nursing. Nursing consists of the giving of care and the co-ordination of care provided by others. Some nurses may wish to use some of the new procedures themselves in order to enhance their nursing, a term used by Helen Passant, a ward sister in Oxford (UK), who practises aromatherapy and some dietary regimens with great enthusiasm. Other nurses may recognise the potential of new therapies for their patients and may build them into the nursing care plan without, necessarily, administering them themselves. Other nurses might prefer the total range of new complementary therapies to be outside their responsibility.

Although there cannot be a definitive answer at present to the appropriate domain of nursing in relation to complementary therapies, it seems prudent to have a flexible attitude to the professional activity of nursing. The role of the nurse depends on many fators which are far from static. The health care setting is changing rapidly and the nursing profession must not only be reactive but, more importantly, pro-active. What constitutes nursing must never be allowed to become a static set of activities engraved on tablets of stone. It is urgent for the nursing profession to demonstrate its unique contribution to the health care of a nation. The Nursing Development Unit in Oxford, pioneered by Dr Alan Pearson, was an all-important initiative. It showed that nurses are uniquely placed to 'move' a patient toward healing and health. In this case, therapeutic nursing was aided by a primary nursing management regimen, but this is neither a necessary nor a sufficient condition. Primary nursing exploits the advantageous position of nurses in relation to their constancy, continuity and the confidence their patients give them. In itself, it does not guarantee therapeutic effects.

Research must play an important part in giving credibility to the practice of therapeutic nursing in the eyes of other disciplines as well as politicians and managers.

The descriptive title of a nurse who practises one of the new therapies may be indicative of the recognition given. The literature shows more therapy-specific than general titles. There are aromatherapists, music therapists, reflexologists, hypnotists etc. Some references to therapeutic nurses and nurse therapists have also been made. The recent history of nursing has shown that many conventinal nursing activities have been taken over by other professionals, such as occupational therapists or physiotherapists. It seems that the omission of 'nurse' in the title may lead to similar developments. However, can a name such as 'therapeutic nurse' really be rationally defended? It seems to lay itself open to much justified ridicule as it implies the possibility of a non-therapeutic nurse. The title 'nurse therapist' indicates either the need for the therapist to be a nurse, a condition which has already been negated, or the possibility of nurses who are not therapists, which undermines the therapeutic effect of conventional nursing.

My preference would be to refrain from seeking new titles simply to connote new activities. Professional nursing should in itself make provision for such an extension. After all, over the last 50 years, the span of my own nursing career, the content of nursing has changed beyond recognition. In the specific context of therapeutic nursing, the healing effect of many conventional nursing activities, such as information giving, has been demonstrated without necessitating the introduction of 'information therapists'. Touch, mentioned earlier, would be another example and 'touch therapist' may not appeal. The original paper which prompted this introduction was closed on a note of optimism, justified by five observations:

1. Questions about the professional nature of nursing are being addressed by committed nurses.
2. Research and evaluation are in progress.
3. The horizons of many nurses are widening.
4. The potential of nursing is being discovered.
5. The urgency of action is being recognised.

This book bears witness to all the above points and adds badly needed knowledge as well as vision.

Holy writ tells us that without vision, people will perish and the nursing profession is not exempt from this sinister prophecy. With vision and the appropriate knowledge to operationalise it, the profession will go from strength to strength and will show the world that nursing, in itself, can contribute significantly to health and healing, the fundamental message of this book.

Lisbeth Hockey PhD, FRCN
Consultant Researcher, Edinburgh

REFERENCES

Altschul, A.T. (1972) *Patient-Nurse Interaction*, University of Edinburgh Department of Nursing Studies, Monograph Number 3. Churchill Livingstone, Edinburgh.
Hobsbaum, E.J. (1962) *The Age of Revolution*, The New American Library, New York.
Hockey, L. (1979) *The Development and Progression of a Long Term Research Programme*, Unpublished PhD Thesis, the City University, London.
Nightingale, F. (1952 edn) *Notes on Nursing* Gerald Duckworth and Co. Ltd., London, p. 15.
Rankin-Box, D.F. (1988) *Complementary Health Therapies: A Guide for Nurses and Caring Professions*, Croom Helm, London.
Redfern, S. and Le May, A. (1986) *Ongoing Study, Nurse–Patient Touch with Elderly Patients*, King's College, London.
Roper, N., Logan, W.W. and Tierney, A.T. (1985) *The Elements of Nursing*, 2nd edn, Churchill Livingstone, Edinburgh.
Wolanin, M. and Phillips, L. (1981) *Confusion: Prevention and Care*, Mosby, St Louis.

Chapter 1

Therapeutic nursing: theory, issues and practice

RICHARD McMAHON

INTRODUCTION

The distinction between the role of the nurse and that of the doctor is frequently described in terms of the 'caring' function of the nurse compared with the 'curative' function of the medical practitioner. The term 'caring' requires clarification, for if it is taken at face value as presented above, it takes on a passive connotation of maintaining or supporting the current health position of a client. Patients for whom all active medical intervention for a cure has been withdrawn are sometimes described as being 'for all nursing care', where the aim is comfort, and little else. Whilst the achieving of comfort for patients is undoubtedly a major nursing function (Wilson-Barnett 1984), many nurses today do not view comfort as an end in itself. Instead, they see the provision of care as a dynamic process which has the patient's health as the objective, which is reflected in such aspects as increased self care ability, self esteem and self determination. Therapeutic nursing is about that dynamic process, which is not merely supportive of the work of others but is potentially a major force in achieving health for the patient.

Current trends in nursing

In the past nursing has frequently been viewed as an adjunct to medicine, as an assistant role, to the latter. For example, 25 years ago one of the items in the final examination for nurse registration involved the correct setting up of a trolley for a medical procedure. This subservience to, and dependence on, the medical profession has arisen out of a number of factors: principally the historical dominance of men over women, the differences in social class between doctors and nurses, and the unique body of (scientific) knowledge of the medical profession (Wright 1985). Oakley (1984) commented that 'if Florence Nightingale had trained her lady pupils in assertiveness rather than obedience, perhaps nurses would be in a different place now'.

Nursing has also been viewed as a custodial service, the legacy of the asylums and workhouses making this particularly pertinent in the fields of mental health and care of elderly people. Even recent research has described the continuation of this, with Evers (1981a and b) describing care in the setting she observed as 'warehousing'. Alfano (1971) identified 34 nursing behaviours and attitudes which make up what she called the ' "caring", task-oriented kind of practice' which she suggested on their own add up to a caretaking service, rather than a professional and healing one. Clearly much nursing practice up to the present day has displayed aspects of the former, rather than the latter.

This lack of a clear healing role, or even desire for such a role in some cases, has led to a potential for what Levi (1980) describes as 'functional redundancy' in nursing. The rise of groups willing to take an active role in mobilising, rehabilitating and nourishing patients led to an early break-up of nursing's monopoly of non-medical health care. Currently, with the move towards doctors' assistants in America and the increasing delegation of 'basic' care for the old and handicapped to care assistants, nursing's remaining role is arguably under threat. It is possible to imagine a future where the activities of qualified nurses in acute hospitals would be almost exclusively related to 'extended' roles, and in other areas such as care of elderly people or in the community the nurse's role would be related to assisting with elimination and the dressing of chronic wounds. The implications of such scenarios have been graphically illustrated by Thomas (1981), who warns that the fragmentation resulting from the allocation of each aspect of care to an 'expert' could lead to the dehumanisation of health care and the isolation of patients.

Alongside this somewhat depressing trend is a movement in nursing to take the initiative and to demonstrate that nurses and nursing have the potential to make a significant contribution to health care. For example, Miller (1985) demonstrated how the traditional practice of 'task allocation' itself led to dependancy among elderly people who were in hospital for more than a month, whereas those receiving individualised care became less dependent. The success of individualised care has been related to the management and individual characteristics of the ward sister (Pembrey 1980, Kitson 1986). Nurses are balancing the emphasis on extended roles with a movement towards expanded roles, that is multi-directional development of nursing-based practices for which qualification as a nurse is a prerequisite. This movement goes hand in hand with the desire to provide holistic care by a united and consistent nursing service. Nurses are recognising that they too are the healers and facilitators who allow the patients to heal themselves. This role is not new, however nurses now have the means through research to demonstrate that nursing is a dynamic force in helping patients towards health. As this research becomes available we have a moral and professional duty to realign our practice along these lines.

Therapeutic nursing, then, is about nurses promoting health and healing for clients under their care. This healing is not 'in spite of' the nursing care, but as a direct result of deliberate nursing decision-making. This chapter provides an introduction to the nursing theory and some of the issues that relate to this idea. It also contains two examples of therapeutic nursing in practice. The chapters that follow examine in greater depth different aspects of therapeutic nursing, and demonstrate some of the research and other work that is being done in this subject.

THERAPEUTIC NURSING IN THEORY

Nursing models

All the principal nursing models view health holistically, and see it as the objective of nursing care. In the past, nurse theorists have considered the therapeutic aspects of nursing from a number of different perspectives. Nightingale strongly believed that good nursing was as responsible for the cure of patients as was the provision of medical preparations. She believed that good nursing involved the manipulation of environmental factors to allow nature to heal the patient. To Nightingale, this included not just the physical but also the interpersonal environment. For example, Nightingale urged the nurse to keep the patient informed as 'apprehension, uncertainty, waiting, expectation, fear of surprise, do a patient more harm than any exertion' (Nightingale 1859).

Few models use the term 'therapeutic' in their vocabulary, however Myra Levine makes a distinction between supportive and therapeutic nursing interventions. To Levine (1973), supportive interventions prevent further deterioration in the health status of patients who are ill, whilst therapeutic interventions are those which promote adaptation and healing, and hence contribute to the restoration of health. Levine is working on a theory of therapeutic intention in nursing (Fawcett 1989). The statements which outline that theory are based on an acknowledgement of the scientific nature of much nursing work, and recognise the nurse's role in such varied activities as the administration of medicines or humanely supporting those who cannot be healed.

Hildegard Peplau emphasises the potential therapeutic value of the nurse–patient relationship, maintaining in particular that 'the nursing process is educative and therapeutic when nurse and patient come to know and respect each other, as persons who are alike, and yet, different, as persons who share in the solution of problems.' (Peplau 1952 p. 9). The themes of the patient knowing the nurse as a person and of the nurse and the patient working in partnership are receiving considerable emphasis today as part of effective nursing practice.

Recent work

The word 'therapy' has been defined in many ways, as has 'nursing'. Hockey (1989) confronted the semantic difficulties of the term 'therapeutic nursing', and suggested that it 'can be described as those nursing activities which result in a movement towards health'. Clearly this has major implications for all those who profess to practise therapeutic nursing. Firstly, the nurse must have a definition of health that is clear and which can be operationalised to form criteria so that the patient's progress can be evaluated. Secondly, the evaluation of care in terms of how well the care was given is inadequate. Care must be principally evaluated through examination of outcomes for the patient; it is only in this way that the effectiveness of the care can be judged. Furthermore, the process of evaluation can be an extremely complex and difficult one for nurses in both practice and research. Finally, those activities and aspects of nursing which have a healing effect require identification and distillation through research.

Nursing as a therapy was discussed in 1986 by McMahon, who considered four areas in which nursing may be considered to be therapeutic, namely the nurse-patient relationship, conventional and unconventional nursing interventions, and patient teaching. 'Conventional' interventions were considered to be those mainly physical treatments that helped to solve such problems as pressure sores, incontinence or feeding difficulties. 'Unconventional' interventions were those based on holism and practices taken from therapies considered to be complementary to medicine, such as kinesiology, massage or aromatherapy. Ersser (1988) also attempted to describe potentially therapeutic elements of nursing, in particular contributing the concepts of the 'therapeutic environment' and of 'providing comfort'. Finally, Muetzel (1988) presented a sophisticated model of the nurse-patient relationship as a therapeutic process, identifying the three elements of partnership, intimacy and reciprocity as key concepts in that process. If these three works are combined the elements of therapeutic nursing may be currently listed as those in Figure 1.1. This list is not intended to be presented as a 'model' of therapeutic nursing – it has inconsistencies and difficulties which will be discussed later – rather it may serve as a framework for categorising points and arguments. It is for that purpose for which it will now be used.

```
*    DEVELOPING – PARTNERSHIP
                – INTIMACY
                – RECIPROCITY
     IN THE NURSE-PATIENT RELATIONSHIP
*    MANIPULATING THE ENVIRONMENT
*    TEACHING
*    PROVIDING COMFORT
*    ADOPTING COMPLEMENTARY HEALTH PRACTICES
*    UTILISING TESTED PHYSICAL INTERVENTIONS
```

Figure 1.1 Therapeutic activities in nursing.

Therapeutic activities in nursing

Six therapeutic activities in nursing are described below. They reflect an underlying belief in the concept of holism (Smuts 1926). Holism implies that the mind and the body are inextricably linked, and that an influence on one may result in change in the other. The recognition of the value of the concept of holism has been widely discussed and accepted by nurses. This assumption that the mind and body should be considered as a whole, and that health is about the well-being of both, seems fundamental to therapeutic nursing. Most, if not all, nursing models describe the individual in social and psychological, as well as physical, terms. Holism provides a wide frame for patient assessment, and for the subsequent attribution of causes to a patient's problems. The activities that might be considered to be therapeutic in nursing reflect an ability for nurses to provide a holistic approach, and even solutions, to these problems.

Developing the nurse–patient relationship

There is much evidence that nurses frequently have interactions with their patients which are not therapeutic; for example Macleod-Clark (1983) demonstrated how many nurses on surgical wards failed to recognise and intervene in relation to patients' psychological discomforts. The need is for a relationship which benefits the patient. Hall (1969) believed that much illness was related to behaviour, and that the nurse could help to move the patient from behaviour that was based on being ill to that which was based on being well through the way she approached and interacted with him. Hall supported the Rogerian method of being non-directive to allow the patient to explore his own feelings and to find solutions to his own problems (Alfano 1985). This has been succinctly described by Peplau who states that 'self-insight operates as an essential tool and as a check in all nurse–patient relationships that are meant to be therapeutic' (Peplau 1952).

Muetzel (1988) links the three concepts of partnership, intimacy and reciprocity which she suggests come together in a therapeutic encounter between the nurse and the patient (Figure 1.2). The interaction between each pair of concepts builds three further concepts of atmosphere, spirit and dynamics. For each of these, Muetzel identifies qualities that characterise that concept. The purpose of these sub-concepts is to demonstrate that it is valid for both the nurse and the patient to benefit from the relationship, that the nurse who is 'self-aware' (or growing towards that goal) has a special contribution to make in the relationship, and that this self awareness is a necessity for the achievement and evaluation of a subjectively therapeutic encounter (Muetzel, personal communication, 1989). It is beyond the scope of this chapter to analyse the model in detail, instead each of the three primary concepts will be briefly examined.

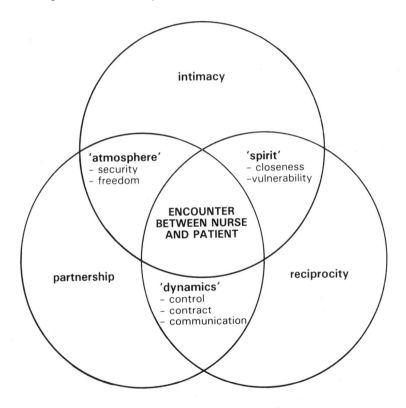

Figure 1.2 Muetzel's model of activities and factors in the therapeutic nurse-patient relationship (adapted from Muetzel 1988).

Partnership is now well established in British nursing literature as a desirable characteristic of the nurse–patient relationship (e.g. Pearson and Vaughan 1986). In its 'Position Statement on Nursing', the Royal College of Nursing stated that:

> Each patient has a right to be a partner in his own care-planning and receive relevant information, support and encouragement from the nurse which will permit him to make informed choices and become involved in his own care.' (RCN 1987)

As partners, both the nurse and the patient have responsibilities to, and expectations of, each other. Intimacy, like partnership, is a two-way process. In the past the nurse was expected to maintain a relationship that did not encourage the expression of feelings by the patient or the nurse. This was justified on the grounds that it was not 'professional' to do so and that nurses could not cope with the stress that would ensue. It would seem to be necessary that the nurse have insight into herself before she can use intimacy safely and effectively (Jourard 1971). Indeed, Muetzel (1988) argues that the ability of the nurse to participate in a therapeutic relationship is reliant on her first having developed as a person and as a member of the nursing team. Hall (1969) and Wharton and Pearson (1988) suggest that the performing of intimate physical care can be a springboard to psychological closeness. Finally, there are elements of reciprocity in both partnership and intimacy. However, as a distinct characteristic reciprocity reflects the belief and value that the nurse-patient relationship may be healing for the nurse as well as the patient. However, the nurse needs to balance her own and the patient's priorities within the relationship against its purpose. Without reciprocity, the nurse-patient relationship almost certainly lacks balance and depth.

Manipulating the environment

The creation of a therapeutic environment can be interpreted to mean the interpersonal as well as the physical environment. The interpersonal environment may be influenced by such factors as the way the nursing delivery system is managed and the belief systems of the nurses. An example of the former is the adoption of primary nursing to maximise contact and continuity between nurse and patient.

In the latter case a ward on which the nurses take their coffee break in the day-room with the patients, drinking from the same cups, has a different ethos and a different environment from a ward where the nurses find the use of the patients' cups distasteful.

However, what constitutes a therapeutic physical environment requires, and is amenable to, further investigation. Should the bath on a care of the elderly ward be one which can be tipped and the side raised to allow easy access for a patient in a wheelchair, or should it be a traditional one into which the patient has to be hoisted, as he will be at home? McMahon (1988) has described how an awareness of the patient's home (preferably acquired by visiting it) can allow the nurse to manipulate the ward environment to simulate problems the patient will have to surmount on discharge.

Health authority planners face a constant dilemma in trying to incorporate the principles of ergonomics and the increasing desire for natural light, air and materials, whilst coming up against pressures of financial restraint. However many health authorities are taking the basic steps of introducing 'no smoking' and healthy eating policies, and many nurses at ward level are working to 'de-institutionalise' their surroundings. There is potential for overlap with the activity of adopting holistic health practices, as the use of essential oils or colours can be environmental manipulations taken from alternative therapies.

Teaching

The investigation of the therapeutic effect of the giving of information by nurses to patients is one of the success stories of nursing research. Davis (1985), having examined much of the research into the subject of pre-operative information-giving, concludes as follows:

> There would seem, therefore, to be a substantial body of evidence demonstrating that patient outcomes, related to a model of stress reduction involving both physiological and

psychological factors, can be significantly influenced by nurses giving pre-operative information.' (Davis 1985)

It is not just pre-operative information giving that has been found to be beneficial to the patient. Other studies have considered the giving of information prior to investigations (Wilson-Barnett 1978) and following myocardial infarction (Thompson 1989) both resulting in beneficial outcomes for the patients.

However, patient teaching has a wider range of interventions than just giving information (Wilson-Barnett 1988). Increasingly nurses are adopting methods that involve the patient participating in the learning process. For example, a person with newly diagnosed diabetes mellitis may progressively practise more of the sequence of actions involved in giving his own insulin, may be encouraged to interpret for himself the implications of his finger-prick blood test and may even be given the experience of mild hypoglycaemia to enable him to recognise his own body's reaction to this.

Providing comfort

Although providing comfort has been identified as one of nursing's key functions (Wilson-Barnett 1984), in many ways this is one of the most controversial of the activities listed. Firstly, the provision of comfort is not always conducive to eliciting a therapeutic effect. For example, the mobilisation of a person following surgery to a fractured neck or femur may be considerably less comfortable than remaining in a bedside chair, however, in terms of regaining independence, the walk may well be more therapeutic. Secondly, it may be argued that comfort is a therapeutic outcome and hence the provision of comfort results from physical interventions, the providing of information, and so on.

The justification for including the provision of comfort as a therapeutic activity lies in the suspicion that these activities, such as giving someone a drink, plumping their pillows or getting an extra blanket, may not be therapeutic merely as a result of their physical effect. It may be that the psychological comfort and warmth of being cared for by another human being, which epitomises nursing (Campbell 1984), does itself aid recovery.

Adopting complementary health practices

At the beginning of this part of the chapter, the comment was made that the concept of holism underlies all these activities. The practising of complementary therapies by nurses would seem to be a logical extension to this idea. Unfortunately, there does seem to be a risk that some nurses interpret the concept of therapeutic nursing as a whole as synonymous with the use of complementary therapies. However, as Newbeck (1986) pointed out, implementing complementary health practices without fundamental change in other aspects of care, such as valueing the nurse-patient relationship, is like trying to ice an uncooked cake. Holism may be practised without necessarily adopting such therapies as massage or reflexology, however the converse is not true.

A number of reservations may be expressed about the use of complementary therapies in nursing. Firstly, at present there is a lack of reliable research evidence demonstrating the efficacy of these practices. This has resulted from a number of factors, such as the lack of research ability amongst complementary therapists regardless of whether they are nurses. A second reservation is that many nurses undertaking these therapies have received minimal training in the practice of that therapy, and as a result are in an untried legal position if anything goes wrong. However, these interventions are now increasingly becoming the subjects of nursing research, and the degree of expertise of some practitioners is extremely high.

Utilising tested physical interventions

The call for nursing to become a research-based occupation has been part of the rhetoric of leaders in nursing for over a decade. The body of research evidence into the efficacy of different physical nursing interventions is expanding rapidly, yet there is considerable evidence that such findings do not readily find their way into nursing practice (Gould 1986). However, until the basis of practice is well understood and articulated, it is difficult to imagine how nurses can deliver care which is consistently therapeutic.

It may be that the desire for therapeutic nursing practice will lead to a change in emphasis away from a milieu in which it is the nurse researchers who beseech practitioners to modify practice as a result of their work. Instead the need for authentic evidence to support practice may result in practitioners governing the direction of knowledge development in the future. Kitson (1987) emphasises that the intuition and 'gut feelings' of practitioners about practice should not be ignored, rather these should be the starting point for tomorrow's research studies. Unfortunately the time when the performance of research is a fundamental component of the practitioner's role is still some time away.

Questioning the elements of therapeutic nursing

The previous pages have been devoted to describing therapeutic activities in nursing. However, although the list presented above is one constructed from a mixture of theoretical and research-based arguments, it has not been tested empirically. Not only does each element in the list require testing, but also combinations of the elements. Similarly, there may be other ways of constructing the list by breaking down and reformulating elements within it. For example, the 'teaching' element could conceivably be absorbed into the activity of the 'nurse-patient relationship'. Similarly, should the idea of taking a holistic approach become included to make a seventh activity or should it remain as an integrated theme running through the others? Questions of this nature are fundamental to the process of clearly identifying and distilling those activities in nursing which are therapeutic. It is only by research into how these elements influence nursing practice, and hence patient outcomes, that nurses can become confident that they know what therapeutic nursing practice actually is.

ISSUES IN THERAPEUTIC NURSING

The location of care

It can be tempting to assume that therapeutic nursing can only occur in areas in which nurses can practise as independent practitioners. However, this is a dangerous assumption, as the vast majority of care takes place in traditional environments which have enormous potential for nurses to orchestrate beneficial outcomes for their patients. The reason for this assumption is that much of the research that can be interpreted as testing therapeutic nursing in practice has come from areas in which nurses have been able to practise independently. Indeed it is the success of that research which has made the concept of therapeutic nursing a reality.

The idea of having areas within health authorities in which nurses have 'control' of the beds, and which allow the aspects of therapeutic nursing to be implemented in a 'safe' environment, have been tested by Pearson et al. (1988a and b). In the two centres or 'nursing units' tested, all the activities identified above were adopted to a large extent. Benefits for patients were demonstrated in terms of levels of independence on discharge, mortality, patient satisfaction and life satisfaction. On the basis of this evidence, the case for opening units in every health authority devoted to 'nursing beds', in which therapeutic nursing can be maximised, is a strong one.

Similarly, clinics run by nurse practitioners have been shown to have favourable results. For example, in a four-year study Curzio et al. (1989) have demonstrated that a blood-pressure clinic run by nurse practitioners can be more effective than a traditional clinic. In the community setting, Stillwell (1988) has investigated the acceptability of a nurse practitioner in general practice and revealed that such a nurse can make a major contribution to the overall health of patients visiting the health centre.

However, regardless of this evidence, the point remains that therapeutic nursing has the potential to be carried out in every ward or other health care setting. The difficulties in implementing and evaluating therapeutic practice can be great in traditional settings where the leader of the multi-disciplinary team is a doctor and where the expectations of the nurses held by all the disciplines involved are at variance. This is a major issue in the success or otherwise of therapeutic nursing.

The value of areas of practice in which nurses can work as independent practitioners is that it is possible to concentrate nursing decision-making and intervention. Furthermore, in such a setting it is easier to try out innovations in practice and to evaluate their effectiveness. Also, many nurses now believe that there are large groups of patients whose needs can be best met in such areas.

Professional boundaries

Patients' problems are often viewed as being the property of the doctor, physiotherapist or other health care worker. This reductionist division of patients' problems into disciplinary areas is a popular but problematic practice. Many health professionals reveal understandable territorial attitudes when they start to feel that nurses may in some way be encroaching on their area of expertise. At the Nursing Development Unit in Oxford, nurses who were seen to assess and intervene with regard to patients' abilities to dress, mobilise and in the care of their relatives following a bereavement, came in for criticism from occupational therapists, physiotherapists and doctors respectively. Indeed, the perception that the patient has separate 'medical' problems, 'nursing' problems and other disciplines' problems is an approach that seems to lead to conflict, due to differing expectations and theoretical frameworks.

In the past nursing has been dominated by the medical model of care which casts the nurse into a supporting role to the doctor. Under that model, doctors subject the patient to a physical or mental examination so as to be able to label the condition and achieve a diagnosis. This is followed, in general, by a pharmacological or surgical treatment which has the goal of curing or suppressing the pathology identified. McFarlane (1980) has promoted the need for a separate nursing model of care in which the person is subjected to a nursing assessment and intervention, with the objective of the patient reaching self-care. Unfortunately, reality is rarely as clear cut as this. Roles frequently overlap and practice is often focused on traditional, rather than theoretical, boundaries.

Consider this example. Suppose that a nursing team helps nature return the skin at the site of a patient's pressure sore to its former integrity by promoting healing through good nursing care. Has there been a cure of that patient's pathology (a 'medical' aim), or have the nurses instead enabled a significant step towards the patient's self-care (a 'nursing' goal) – or have they effectively done both? It would seem that it is not the outcome of the care (in this case, the healed sore) so much as the means used to achieve it (turning and the applying of dressings) which identifies this as a nursing rather than a medical outcome.

Therefore, much of the disharmony between different health care occupations seems to result from the attempt to label physical, mental and even social conditions as being 'nursing', 'medical' or any other discipline's problems, with that disharmony inevitably being to the detriment of the patient and the wider health care service. The solution to this disharmony may lie in an approach which focuses on the identification and labelling of *patient's* problems or needs which may be amenable to the interventions of nurses, doctors or other health care workers either alone, or more probably, in combination. Consider a different example: it has been shown that the provision of pre-operative information-giving can result in less post-operative pain (e.g. Hayward 1975). This effect does not, however, negate the use of all pharmacological analgesia for the patient who has returned from the operating theatre; good care is the result of combining the two, not substituting one with the other.

Therapeutic nursing, then, is about achieving beneficial outcomes for people by applying nursing interventions to problems designated as being those of the patient rather than the property of one discipline or another. Those interventions should be applied in a way that acknowledges and complements the work of other therapists with due regard for the goals and individuality of the patient. If the whole multidisciplinary team recognises this, a certain amount of harmony can be achieved between nursing and other therapies.

The need to be pro-active

The extent to which, for much of its history, nursing has been described as a custodial service has already been described. It would seem, then, that one of the first steps towards therapeutic nursing is that nurses themselves actually recognise that they have the ability, authority and even a duty to intervene positively to solve patients' problems. This may not only appear to be stating the obvious, but also describing what nurses instinctively do every day. However, research examining nurse to nurse communication indicated that on some of the wards observed nurses seemed to have little awareness that they were discussing problems to which nursing may have been able to provide a solution (McMahon, forthcoming). In some cases, where problems were identified in the nurses' handover for which nursing does have established and proven interventions to offer, these were noted for referral to the doctor or other health care worker for them to deal with. On other occasions, a problem such as a patient's incontinence was reported during the handover, but was apparently taken as a 'fait accompli', and as a result provoked no discussion amongst the nurses whatsoever. Such observations are indicative of an approach which is not therapeutic, and under such circumstances it is not surprising that other disciplines take on the care for problems for which nurses show no awareness of having something positive to offer. Levine has been reported as commenting that nurses should conceptualise about patients and their problems in a way similar to doctors (Profile 1974). It may well be that discussing, selecting and refining nursing interventions through consultation at a collegial level with other nurses is another factor which facilitates therapeutic nursing.

Nurses must be wary of passivity in their approach, and should not regard themselves only as instruments of other therapists, or caretakers whilst waiting for other disciplines to heal the patient. The realisation that they can become highly significant in the patient's return to health is the first step to nurses becoming pro-active in care.

The ability to take risks

The need for strength and courage amongst those who practise therapeutic nursing results in part from the fact that all who profess to prescribe care must be accountable, and that effective prescribing involves an element of risk-taking.

Gilchrist (1987) has illustrated some of the difficulties requiring risk-taking in a care of the elderly setting. As 23% of patients who came to his ward did so following a fall, the likelihood of further falls on the ward was high. However, this did not negate the need to rehabilitate those patients by encouraging them to mobilise again, even though in some cases a further fall could have resulted in the loss of sufficient functional ability, or confidence, to go home.

Unfortunately nurses are rarely taught how to take a risk, and in fact many nurses are trained in such a way as to minimise any danger in what they do, both for the patients and for themselves. Yet if nurses are to be pro-active, to prescribe nursing care that is dynamic and which benefits the lives of patients, then they must accept the risk of failure and any consequent legal or professional investigation. Carson (1988) provided an assessment strategy (Figure 1.3) which described a method for helping nurses to make a decision when presented with a situation which required the taking of a risk. Carson distinguishes between taking a gamble (something that is done voluntarily and which has a high chance of failure), a risk (which involves weighing pros and cons) and facing a dilemma (when a decision has to be made between choices which may each have benefits and possibilities of harm). Carson emphasises the need to weigh benefits against possibilities of harm, and acknowledges that in some cases nurses have a duty to take a risk, for example in condoning the discharge of one patient because another patient who is seriously ill needs the bed. Carson makes it clear that the inclusion and consent of the patient in taking a risk is a strong buttress with which to support the final decision.

1.   Analyse whether the proposed action is best described as a gamble, a risk or a dilemma.
2.   List all the possible kinds of benefits, for the patient, of acting.
3.   List all the possible kinds of benefits, and knock-on benefits, for other people.
4.   Analyse the likelihood of each of these benefits occurring.
5.   Manipulate the risk by taking steps to make the benefits more likely to occur.
6.   List all the possible kinds of harm, to the patient, of acting.
7.   List all the possible kinds of harm, and knock-on harms, to other people.
8.   Analyse the likelihood of each of these harms occurring.
9.   Manipulate the risk by taking steps to reduce the likelihood of the harms occurring.
10. List duties to risk.
11. Obtain the patient's informed consent.
12. Obtain the informed agreement of colleagues.
13. Assess whether 'the risk' should be taken.

Figure 1.3 Assessment strategy for taking risks with patients (from Carson 1988, with permission from Austen Cornish Publishing).

THERAPEUTIC NURSING IN PRACTICE

So far, this chapter has addressed mainly theoretical issues. However, therapeutic nursing is about clinical practice, and requires nurses who are well prepared, and who are able to analyse and evaluate their practice. Two examples of therapeutic nursing in practice are given below to illustrate how the concepts can be operationalised.

Example 1

Consider a nurse caring for a group of patients on a ward at night. Night nursing has been described as a 'reactive and demand-led service' (DHSS 1987). By contrast, the effective night nurse who achieves beneficial outcomes for her patients, and is hence giving therapeutic care, is pro-active rather than reactive. She does not regard sleeplessness as a 'medical' problem, instead she views it as one of the patient's problems that the nurse can help to solve. As a first step she actively settles each of the patients. To 'actively settle' the patients, the nurse has to ensure consciously that each patient is as comfortable as possible. This may involve, for example, the giving of adequate analgesia, helping the patient to void his bladder and helping him to achieve a comfortable position in the bed. The therapeutic night nurse also aims to create a therapeutic environment. This is on the one hand the physical environment, requiring an awareness of the need to use hushed voices and to reduce the volume of the television or the telephone bell, and on the other the patient's interpersonal environment. This is achieved by giving information that reassures the patient, for example that there is always a nurse on the ward during the night and telling him how to summon the nurse and not to be afraid to do so. The way the nurse communicates that message tells the patient whether the nurse really means this or not. The relationship between the night nurse and the patient can exhibit partnership in that the nurse negotiates with the patient what time he likes to retire in the evening and what time he likes to rise.

Where the patient suffers insomnia due to anxiety or depression, the nurse can use his or her self therapeutically, which requires self-disclosure rather than the adopting of the so-called 'professional' front. This two-way openness between nurse and patient reflects the aspect of intimacy. In such a situation, it is not necessarily inappropriate that the nurse should express her own anxieties and feelings, and this can lead the patient to a state of interdependence and reciprocity with the nurse.

Where the nurse assesses that the patient's sleeplessness is due to stress, being pro-active might involve performing a head or neck massage, or teaching the patient a progressive relaxation exercise. By having knowledge of the benzodiazepines the nurse is able to advise the patient on the advantages and disadvantages of commencing or continuing these drugs. From awareness of research, the nurse does not encourage all patients to have a milky drink on retiring as she knows that such beverages tend only to help those who are accustomed to having them as part of their usual nightly routine – the drinks actually delaying sleep for those who do not usually have them (Brezinova and Oswald 1972, Adam 1980). Finally, the nurse takes a risk in not waking one of the patients at 6 a.m. to take his blood pressure, having decided with the patient that he would benefit most from sleeping until 8 a.m. and having it taken then.

Example 2

Imagine a nurse assessing Mrs Brown (a genuine patient whose name has been changed), who has an exuding ulcer extending around her leg and which has broken down following recent skin grafting. When confronted with a patient with a break in the integrity of her skin, it is very easy to assess the wound and not the person. The therapeutic nurse assesses the patient holistically: she not only assesses the size, colour, topographical appearance, exudate and odour of the wound, and the condition of the surrounding skin, but also interviews Mrs Brown and scrutinises her previous nursing and medical records. In this case, this reveals a multitude of factors relevant to the healing potential for the wound (Figure 1.4). Mrs Brown has suffered from leg ulcers from the age of 30. The problem with the venous return in her legs is clearly a hereditary one as Mrs Brown has revealed that her sister had also had severe ulceration of her legs, to the extent that she had undergone an amputation and unfortunately subsequently died. Mrs Brown herself has had three operations on the veins in her legs, and has had her current ulcer for several years. She is a known diabetic, controlled on oral hypoglycaemics, and her blood chemistry evaluations reveal her to be anaemic and show that her serum albumen is only 32 g/l, when the normal range is 35–50 g/l. Mrs Brown comes across as an angry person, and although she wants her ulcer to heal, she considers the pain that it causes her to be her main problem. Furthermore, Mrs Brown blames the district nurses for the eventual failure of her skin graft. Later during her stay, she explains that she does not get on well with her husband, who she describes as a 'good for nothing', and says that he throws crockery at her when he gets in a temper.

Factor	Nursing implications
Aetiology, appearance, size, smell, location of ulcer.	Choice of dressing. Other nursing interventions (e.g. elevation, compression, exercise etc.)
History of vein surgery and recurrent ulcers since age 30 (now aged over 80).	Poor prognosis for healing of ulcer.
Death of sister following amputation of leg.	Anxiety and reluctance to agree to amputation of own leg. Reactive depression.
Diabetes mellitus.	Probably poor healing potential. Potential ineffective and arterial problems. Dietary considerations and assessment of knowledge base.
Anaemia and low serum protein.	Rest and dietary considerations.
Anger and irritability associated with severe pain.	The need to break the 'vicious circle'. Analgesia, relaxation. Choice of dressing.
Blame for failure of graft placed with district nurses.	Possible lack of trust and confidence in ward nurses. Implications for discharge.
Unhappy home situation.	Possible poor compliance with treatment to postpone discharge

Figure 1.4 The nursing implications for the care of Mrs Brown based on factors arising from a holistic assessment.

Clearly, the salient question for the therapeutic nurse is not 'what dressing shall we apply to this ulcer?', but 'how shall we care for Mrs Brown?'

From the assessment, the nurse realises that the chances of healing Mrs Brown's ulcer are slim. However, she can still achieve beneficial outcomes for her, such as reducing her pain, anxiety, exudate and lethargy, and also help her to come to terms with the prospect of an amputation. From her knowledge of venous leg ulcers, the nurse knows that manipulating the environment so that Mrs Brown can keep her legs elevated in the bed will reduce the exudate (Ryan 1987). However, as her compliance is poor, the nurse spends much time teaching Mrs Brown about leg ulcers, and in partnership with her produces a 'legs up' plan, which is seen as a contract between the nurse and the patient (Ciske 1979). The nurse also uses aromatherapy oils to create a pleasant atmosphere in Mrs Brown's room, particularly when the leg is being dressed. By getting 'close' to Mrs Brown, the nurse is able to find out the reason for Mrs Brown's poor compliance, namely her reluctance to return home to her husband. Finally, by using the tested intervention of dressing the ulcer with a hydrocolloid dressing, the nurse is able to provide comfort as this has been shown considerably to reduce the pain from leg ulcers (Ryan et al. 1985, van Rijswijk et al. 1985).

These two examples were selected so as to give a 'feel' for the concept of therapeutic nursing. Clearly, in these examples the therapeutic nurse draws on many of the activities identified in this chapter, and confronts some of the issues that have been discussed. They help to demonstrate that by careful assessment the pro-active nurse is able to control the situation and turn it to the benefit of his or her patients, rather than being controlled by it herself.

CONCLUSION

This chapter has provided an introduction to the concepts behind the idea of nursing as a therapy. It has identified why nursing has often been far from therapeutic in the past, and has traced the idea from Florence Nightingale to the present day. In presenting a list of activities that can make nursing practice benefit patients, the aim was to provide a framework for analysis and discussion and not to present a definitive model or theory.

In highlighting activities that nurses do, there are aspects of therapeutic nursing that this chapter has not addressed. For example, how nurses can be prepared to function at this level is an issue which requires careful consideration. Similarly, it can be suggested that simply practising in a way that adopts the activities presented in this chapter is only half way to therapeutic practice. Nurses need to be able constantly to analyse and evaluate their work, in such a way as to allow them to formulate new and creative solutions to problems presented by patients who are all different, and who are never quite as the textbooks portray them. The cultivation of these skills is a major challenge. Other issues include how to create an environment which fosters therapeutic practice, and whether the highly problem-orientated approach taken in this chapter is necessarily always the most effective for creating beneficial outcomes for patients. These and other issues are addressed in the chapters that follow.

Therapeutic nursing is about nurses using their creativity to intervene positively to assist the patient in his or her quest for health. It relies on nurses being committed to clinical practice, and on nurse managers, educators and researchers providing the necessary environment and knowledge for that practice to be effective. The widespread adoption of the concept of nursing as a therapy could mark the start of a new era characterised by improved care for patients.

REFERENCES

Adam, K. (1980) 'Dietary habits and sleep after bedtime food drinks', *Sleep*, **3** 47–58.
Alfano, G.J. (1971) 'Healing or caretaking – which will it be?' *Nursing Clinics of North America*, **6**(2), 273–80.
Alfano, G. (1985) 'Whom do you care for?', *Nursing Practice*, **1**(1) 28–31.
Brezinova, V. and Oswald, I. (1972) 'Sleep after a bedtime beverage', *British Medical Journal*, **2**(5811), 431–3.
Campbell, A.V. (1984) *Moderated Love: A Theology of Professional Care*, SPCK, London.
Carson, D. (1988) 'Taking risks with patients – your assessment strategy', *The Professional Nurse*, **3**(7), 247–50.
Cassee, E. (1975) 'Therapeutic behaviour, hospital culture and

communication', in Cox, C. and Mead, A. (eds) *A Sociology of Medical Practice*, Collier-Macmillan, London.

Ciske, K.L. (1979) 'Accountability – the essence of primary nursing', *American Journal of Nursing*, **79**(5), 890–4.

Curzio, J.L., Reid, J.L., Rubin, P.C., Elliott, H.L. and Kennedy, S.S. (1989) *A Comparison of Care of the Hypertensive Patient: Nurse Practitioner vs. Traditional Medical Care*, RCN Research Society Annual Conference, Swansea.

Davis, B. (1985) 'The clinical effect of interpersonal skills: the implementation of pre-operative information giving', in Kagan, C.M. (ed.) *Interpersonal Skills in Nursing*, Croom Helm, London.

Department of Health and Social Security (1987) *Study of Night Nursing Services*, HMSO, London.

Ersser, S. (1988) 'Nursing Beds and Nursing Therapy' in Pearson, A. (ed.) *Primary Nursing: Nursing in the Burford and Oxford Nursing Development Units*, Croom Helm, London.

Evers, H.K. (1981a) 'Care or custody? The experience of women patients in long-stay geriatric wards', in Hutter, B. and Williams, G. (eds) *Controlling Women: The Normal and the Deviant*, Croom Helm, London.

Evers, H.K. (1981b) 'Tender loving care? Patients and nurses in geriatric wards', in Copp, L.A. (ed.) *Recent Advances in Nursing 2: Care of the Ageing*, Churchill Livingstone, Edinburgh.

Fawcett, J. (1989) *Analysis and Evaluation of Conceptual Models of Nursing. (2nd edn)*, F.A. Davis Co., Philadelphia.

Gilchrist, B. (1987) 'Taking risks for quality', *Geriatric Nursing and Home Care*, **7**(11) 24–6.

Gould, D. (1986) 'Pressure sore prevention and treatment: an example of nurses' failure to implement research findings', *Journal of Advanced Nursing*, **11**(4) 389–94.

Kitson, A.L. (1986) 'Indicators of quality in nursing care – an alternative approach', *Journal of Advanced Nursing*, **11**(2), 33–144.

Kitson, A.L. (1987) 'Raising standards of clinical practice – the fundamental issue of effective nursing practice', *Journal of Advanced Nursing*, **12**(3), 321–9.

Hall, L. (1969) 'The Loeb Center for Nursing and Rehabilitation, Montefiore Hospital and Medical Center, Bronx, New York', *International Journal of Nursing Studies*, **6** 81–97.

Hayward, J. (1975) *Information – A prescription against pain*, Royal College of Nursing, London.

Hockey, L. (1989) 'Therapeutic nursing: Its development and debut', Oxford, Therapeutic Nursing Conference (unpublished paper).

Jourard, S. (1971) *The Transparent Self*, Van Nostrand, New Jersey.

Levi, M. (1980) 'Functional redundancy and the process of professionalization: the case of registered nurses in the United States', *Journal of Health Politics, Policy and Law*, **5**(2), 333–53.

Levine, M.E. (1973) *Introduction to Clinical Nursing* (2nd edn) F.A. Davis Co., Philadelphia.

Macleod-Clark, J. (1983) 'Nurse-patient communication – an analysis of conversations from surgical wards', in Wilson-Barnet, J. (ed.) *Nursing Research: Ten Studies in Patient Care*, John Wiley, Winchester.

McFarlane, J.K. (1980) *The Multi-Disciplinary Team*, King's Fund, London.

McMahon, R.A. (1986) 'Nursing as a therapy', *The Professional Nurse*, 1(10), 270–2.

McMahon, R.A. (1988) 'Discharge planning: home truths', *Geriatric Nursing and Home Care*, 8(9), 16–17.

McMahon, R.A. (1990) 'Power and collegial relations among nurses on wards adopting primary nursing and hierarchical ward management structures, *Journal of Advanced Nursing*, 15(2), 232–9.

Miller, A. (1985) 'Nurse/patient dependancy – is it Iatrogenic?' *Journal of Advanced Nursing*, 10(1), 63–70.

Muetzel, P. (1988) Therapeutic nursing in Pearson, A. (ed.) *Primary Nursing: Nursing in the Burford and Oxford Nursing Development Units*, Croom Helm, London.

Newbeck, I. (1986) 'How holistic therapies can be used in nursing', Second Holistic Nursing Conference, City University, London.

Nightingale, F. (1859) (republished 1980) *Notes on Nursing*, Churchill Livingstone, Edinburgh.

Oakley, A. (1984) 'The importance of being a nurse', *Nursing Times*, 80(50), 24–7.

Pearson, A., Durand, I., and Punton, S. (1988a) 'The feasibility and effectiveness of nursing beds', *Nursing Times*, 84(9), 48–50.

Pearson, A., Durand, I., and Punton, S. (1988b) *Therapeutic Nursing: an Evaluation of an Experimental Nursing Unit in the British National Services*, research report, Oxfordshire Health Authority.

Pearson, A. and Vaughan, B. (1986) *Nursing Models for Practice*, Heinemann, London.

Pembrey, S.M. (1980) *The Ward Sister – Key to Nursing*, Royal College of Nursing, London.

Peplau, H. (1952) *Interpersonal Relations in Nursing*, G.P. Putnam's Sons, New York.

Profile (1974) Myra E. Levie, RN, MS *Nursing '74*, 5 p. 70.

Ryan, T.J., Given, H.F., Murphy, J.J., Rope-Ross, M. and Byrnes, G. (1985) 'The use of a new occlusive dressing in the management of venous stasis ulceration' in Ryan, T.J. (ed), *An Environment for Healing: the Role of Occlusion*, Royal Society of Medicine, London.

Stillwell, B. (1988) 'Patient's attitudes to the availability of a nurse practitioner in general practice', in Bowling, A. and Stillwell, B. *The Nurse in Family Practice*, Scutari Marketings, London.

Ryan, T.J. (1987) *The Management of Leg Ulcers* (2nd edn) Oxford University Press, Oxford.

Smuts, J.C. (1926) *Holism and Evolution* Macmillan, New York.

Thomas, S.P. (1981) 'The advantures of Joey in Patientland: a futuristic fantasy', *Nursing Forum*, 19, 351–7.

Thompson, D.R. (1989) 'A randomized controlled trial of in-hospital nursing support for first-time myocardial infarction patients and their partners: effects on anxiety and depression', *Journal of Advanced Nursing*, **14**(4), 291–7.

Van Rijswijk, L., Brown, D., Friedman, S., Degreef, H., Roed-Petersen, J., Borglund, E., Sayag, J., Beylot, C. and Daniel Su, W.P. (1985) 'Multicenter clinical evaluation of a hydrocolloid dressing for leg ulcers', *Cutis* **35** 173–6.

Wharton, A. and Pearson, A. (1988) 'Nursing and intimate physical care: the key to therapeutic nursing', in Pearson, A. (ed.) *Primary Nursing: Nursing in the Burford and Oxford Nursing Development Units*, Croom Helm, London.

Wilson-Barnett, J. (1978) 'Patients' emotional response to barium X-rays', *Journal of Advanced Nursing*, **3**(1), 37–45.

Wilson-Barnett, J. (1984) *Key functions in nursing: The Fourth Winifred Raphael Memorial Lecture*, Royal College of Nursing, London.

Wilson-Barnett, J. (1988) 'Patient teaching or patient counselling?', *Journal of Advanced Nursing*, **13**(2), 215–22.

Wright, S. (1985) 'New nurses: new boundaries', *Nursing Practice*, **1**(1), 32–9.

Chapter 2

Reflection and the evaluation of experience: prerequisites for therapeutic practice

JEAN POWELL

The title of this chapter is a little presumptuous and reflects the personal belief of the author. This is, however, supported by the work of writers and researchers in the field of professional practice (Boud and Griffin 1987, Schon 1983, Marsick 1987) but is not yet as universally accepted as the statement suggests. The chapter will discuss the concept of reflection, experiential learning and the evaluation of experience and argue that these are indeed essential for therapeutic practice in nursing.

Therapeutic practice can be simply defined as practice where the nurse has made a positive difference to a patient's or client's health state, and where he or she is aware of how and why this positive difference occurred. In addition there should be awareness of the reasons behind a failure to achieve any positive difference in health state. The nature of nursing practice is also relevant here and warrants further discussion.

NURSING PRACTICE

Nursing is a complex and dynamic activity which has been defined in many different ways. Some definitions are visionary and entirely abstract such as:

nursing is a responsible searching, transactional relationship whose meaningfulness demands conceptualization founded on a nurse's existential awareness of self and of the other (Paterson and Zderad 1988).

Others are more down to earth such as:

the unique function of the nurse is to assist the individual, sick or well, in the performance of those activities contributing to health or its recovery (or to peaceful death) that he would perform unaided if he had the necessary strength, will or knowledge. And to do this in such a way as to help him gain independence as rapidly as possible (Harmer and Henderson 1955).

The latter is more likely to appeal to British nurses, as can be seen by the number of times it is quoted in assignments submitted by nurses on courses ranging from initial nurse education to English National Board (ENB) and diploma/degree courses. This may be because it is a practical definition describing what nurses do rather than what nursing is.

Nurses are doers and this doing is highly valued in the culture of the nursing world. The socialisation of new entrants into this world is ensured by the requirement that learner nurses are also a major part of the workforce. While much teaching does go on in clinical areas, the prime requirement of the ward staff is that learners be able to carry out the nursing work, from bedbaths and simple technical tasks, such as temperature and blood pressure measurement, to nursing assessments for care. Although supervision is explicitly expected, it is obvious that it cannot be carried out while learners are also workers, other than at the most superficial level i.e. has the task allocated been adequately carried out?

This means that work is emphasised over learning, and that where teaching takes place, the learning resulting from this tends to relate to discrete tasks, with little development of a critical approach. As Procter (1989) has pointed out in her research into the effects of using a mainly transient workforce (learner nurses) on nursing care:

The current organization of nursing work at ward level does not promote a utilization of nursing knowledge by qualified nurses to resolve the dilemmas and ambiguities inherent in patient care.

The implications are that not only is the bulk of nursing care being given by untrained and transient workers, but that this very element militates against qualified staff developing their knowledge base through either innovation or experience. Some nurses undoubtedly overcome the barriers to reach Benner's 'expert' level but these would appear to be the exception rather than the rule. Benner drew her examples of expert care from

'outstanding clinical situations where the nurse learned something about her practice or made a significant contribution to a patient's welfare' (Benner 1984).

The need for nurses to associate excellence in practice with learning from practice is a key premiss here. This is an issue also developed by Schon (1983) although there are fundamental differences between his work and Benner's in that she emphasises the need to consider intuitive feelings while Schon emphasises the use of experience as a kind of individual research through reflection. 'Reflection gives rise to on the spot experiment' (Schon 1987). Schon's work will be discussed more thoroughly later in this chapter.

The nature of professional nursing practice seems to have several key elements, one being the need for a sound knowledge base, and another the ability to understand exactly what a health problem or disability means to the person. This might be called empathy, but this term seems rather vague. What is implied here is that the nurse may need to reframe the problem depending on the individual. The problem may superficially appear the same e.g. stiff, painful knee and hip joints in an arthritic patient. Assuming that this is not amenable to further medical or paramedical intervention, the problem then is what effect this has on the patient's life and how it makes him or her feel.

This reframing of a problem will not only relate to the knowledge and experience of the nurse and the individuality of the patient, but also to the way the practitioner feels about the problem. Some aspects of a problem will provoke stronger feelings than others, and the feelings may be positive or negative. The positive feelings may only need to be acknowledged but negative ones may need discussing to determine their significance. This is important as it may affect the learning process and future practice. Much work has been done on this by Boud and Griffin (1987).

This implies the ability to communicate well with others and to build up effective relationships so that health problems can be alleviated. The nature of the relationship between nurse and patient or client is crucial here, with the nurse recognising that it is the patient who makes the decisions, except in very special circumstances, such as unconsciousness. This can be difficult in practice, where the reality of a busy ward with the many demands on the nurse's time, make it easy for the nurse to take a dominant role.

Being able to build on the knowledge base by both conventional and experiential means must also be a key factor in sound practice. The ever-changing nature of nursing and the individuality of the situations within nursing mean that those who do not learn are left behind, and are likely to be increasingly ineffective as carers, as well as possibly unfulfilled and dissatisfied employees.

An awareness of moral issues, and the basic tools to analyse and clarify these, are a priority for professional practitioners of any kind. For nurses, because of the vulnerability of the patient/client groups, this is of prime importance. Unfortunately at present the development of sensitivity to moral issues, and the teaching of the necessary skills, are not given priority within the curriculum and in many cases are relegated to one or two hours, often taught by a nurse tutor who may be sensitive to the issues but rarely has the ability to impart the skills needed.

EXPERIENTIAL LEARNING AND REFLECTION

Much of the interest in experiential learning developed from both education, through Dewey, and the social sciences, with Lewin's (1935) work in the United States and Habermas' (1971) in Germany. Dewey (1933) produced a problem-solving design, which was an early model of the actual experience of learning. He reasoned that all thinking had its origins in problematic situations, and that this thinking is an enabling device for interaction between the individual and his environment. He defined problematic situations as being those which cannot be resolved by the use of prior solutions. This is very similar to Schon's view of the problems faced by professionals and the development of strategies for solving these (Schon 1983).

Dewey also emphasised the active nature of learning, where an experience is in two parts, firstly, the undergoing of the experience, and secondly, the thought and consideration of what this experience meant. He wrote that we do not 'learn by doing' . . . 'we learn by doing and realising what came of what we did' (Dewey 1929, p. 367). This type of learning offers developmental and growth potential which exceeds the requirements of the immediate situation, and which cannot only be transferred to other situations, but, because of this growth potential, may enable this further experience to be of greater significance.

Other writers have produced problem solving models (Urban and Ford 1971, Garry and Kingsley 1970, Garrison 1964, among others). Some have highlighted the creative aspects of this, such as Osborne (1953) who developed a seven-stage model on the same lines as Dewey, but who added the concept of 'incubation', the stage where the halting of active reasoning appears to allow a spontaneous generation of a solution to the problem.

If Dewey was undoubtedly a major influence on experiential learning, producing new insights from the field of education, particularly with those books published in 1916, 1929 and 1938, an equally important influence came from Lewin's work in the field of social science. This work was mainly carried out in the 1940s and provided further insights into experiential learning. Lewis (1935) refers to the 'life space' of the individual, the interaction of the complexity of factors influencing the context in which learning takes place. This individual interaction affects the development of a learning style that will enable the individual to know, explain and cope with his world and the experiences it provides.

At around the same time, Habermas, one of the Frankfurt school of social philosophers, proposed that knowledge was generated in three separate ways: through the area of work which he saw as comprising the aspects where control and manipulation of the environment were occurring; through the practical area where interaction would assist in interpreting the situations and identifying conditions for furtherance of this; and through the emancipatory area which is concerned with self exploration, leading to self knowledge and reflection (Habermas, cited in Mezirow 1981). This important foundation was further advanced by the work of Kolb and Fry (1975) in their exposition of an experiential learning model with concrete experience followed by observations and reflections, leading to the formation of abstract concepts and generalisations, which could then be used to test implications of the concepts in new situations. This work has since been developed more fully by Kolb (1984). The emergence of the model was a rigorous attempt to understand the dynamics of the learning process in experiential learning.

Kolb and Fry sought to clarify four aspects of experiential learning:

1. the integration of the cognitive and socio-economic perspectives on learning;
2. the role of individual differences in learning style;
3. the concept of growth and development inherent in the experiential learning model;
4. a model of learning environments that is commensurate with the experiential learning process (Kolb and Fry 1975).

The model is a cyclical one which is designed to be consistent with both the structure of cognition and also with growth and development. One of its major features was the emphasis on learning styles and their individuality. Kolb and Fry defined four main styles: convergent, divergent, assimilating and accommodating. While they recognise that these styles are overlapping and that within each is a great diversity and complexity, they do stress the opposition of reflection and action, claiming that each inhibits the other (1975).

This separation of reflection and action has led to general acceptance of the view of reflection and action as not only very different but as inhibitors of each other. Schon's work on reflective practice (1983) is the first to dispute this and to promote the idea of reflection-in-action, assisting both the action and learning from it. This will be discussed more thoroughly later in this work.

The Kolb and Fry learning cycle is, however, extremely important in that it represents a method of separating the learning occurring from experience into various elements which can then be studied. The cycle itself is simplistic and it can be seen that, for example, reflection must also occur at the third stage of formulating concepts (Jarvis and Gibson 1985), but this is possibly more of an aid to examination of the various aspects than a defect.

Reflection in its relation to experiential learning and hence to therapeutic practice is the main concern of this chapter and therefore it is important to examine more directly the whole concept of reflection. Reflection in learning is not a new idea, indeed it is akin to Aristotle's concept of deliberation (Elliot 1983). Dewey also discussed the problems in 'forming habits of reflective thought' (Dewey 1933), and he later defined reflective thought as:

> 'Active, persistent and careful consideration of any belief or support form of knowledge in the light of the grounds that support it, and further conclusions to which it leads . . . it includes a conscious and voluntary effort to establish belief upon a firm basis of evidence and rationality' (Dewey 1933).

Dewey has undoubtedly provided a great deal of the foundation for current thinking on reflection and learning, although the present emphasis appears to be more on the creativity and affective elements of reflection rather than the rationality of it as a process. This can be seen, for example, in the work of Boyd and Fales (1983) who see reflective learning emphasising 'the self as the source of learning and . . . therefore inherently an individual and ipsative process'. They define reflection as:

> 'the process of creating and clarifying the meaning of experience (present or past) in terms of self (self in relation to self and self in relation to the world)'

and further state that:

> 'the outcome of the process is a changed conceptual perspective' (Boyd and Fales 1983).

They feel that reflection is a natural process used spontaneously by many people and as such is not a new concept, but that its present significance lies in reflection as a 'paradigm shift' in 'professional learning from experience, personal growth . . . both in professionals' own continuing learning, and in facilitating the learning and growth of their clients'. A further aspect of their work is the emphasis on consciousness-raising and of their description of beginning reflection as a sense of 'inner discomfort' (ibid). Consciousness-raising echoes Freire's work and his concept of conscientisation with its links to reflection. Similar ideas are promoted by Goldstein (1981) in his discussion of discrimination learning which he conceives as being:

> primarily focussed on the perceptual functions of consciousness and attention to enable the individual to become more sensitive and responsive to these aspects of his experience that, for some reason, remain obscure.

Boud, working with Keogh and Walker (1985), has produced a model for promoting reflection in learning where they define reflection as:

> a generic term for those intellectual and affective activities in which individuals engage to explore their experiences in order to lead to new understandings and appreciations.'
> (1985)

This model emphasises the affective aspects of learning and how these may facilitate or hinder reflection. Feelings throughout the experience are of fundamental importance here, and Boud also highlights the relationship of these to past experiences.

This importance given to the affective nature of learning also emphasises its individuality, and therefore the control must always be with the learner, with the teacher acting as facilitator, with access only to such information as the learner wishes him to have (Boud 1985). This is similarly emphasised in Knowles' work, where he places great stress on the building up of trust between learner and teacher.

Knowles acknowledges the control vested in the learner further in his discussions on andragogy, with the involvement of the learner in diagnosing his own needs and planning of learning contracts to meet those needs. Experiential learning is a key component of andragogy and Knowles highlights the vast range of adult learners' experience, and therefore the complexity of the effects of this on learning experiences and the essential individuality of these (Knowles 1985). While andragogy is not a theory of experiential learning *per se*, it has undoubtedly added much to present-day thinking on and practice of this, and also to the thinking on and practice of reflection. His use of learning contracts means they cannot be effective without this reflection and careful consideration at all stages (Knowles 1985).

Further ideas on reflection have been put forward by Kemmis (1985) to suggest that reflection is a social rather than an individual process. This is based on the interesting premise that:

> 'the fruits of reflection-action have their meaning and significance in a social world, in which others understand us through our actions (including our utterances) and, as Wittgenstein (1974) showed, in which we can invest meaning in our actions only by reference to the forms of life we share with others.' (1985)

Kemmis separated reflection into three different but parallel forms: problem solving, practical deliberation and speculative thought. The last is closely linked to the Habermas (1971) concept of initial reflection. Each of the three forms are action-orienting and therefore Kemmis strongly promotes the concept of reflection as both political and ideological. Although Kemmis does not refer to Freire's writings in his work, there would appear to be strong links between them.

Other writers have related reflection purely to post action thinking (Clarke 1985, Shotter 1974). While this is valuable it is only a part of the complex process of reflection and more critical studies such as Habermas, whose contribution to experiential learning was discussed earlier in this chapter, and Mezirow are therefore more relevant to the discussion here.

Habermas (1971) proposed that reflection is always intentional and talked of 'critical intent'. Mezirow has largely built on the work of Habermas but analysed reflection in greater detail and used it to clarify his concept of learning as 'perspective transformation'. Mezirow (1981) classifies reflection as having seven forms which act as a type of hierarchy of reflective activity. This begins with reflectivity, where there is awareness of specific perception, meaning or behaviour or of limits regarding these. Affective reflectivity is becoming aware of feelings with regard to reflectivity, while discriminant reflectivity assesses the effectiveness of perceptions, thoughts, actions and habits. Judgmental reflectivity is closely related to this in that it is concerned with awareness of value judgements regarding perception, thought, actions and habits.

These four can be seen to be on a different level to the last three which are particularly concerned with perspective transformation. They are all concerned with critical thought rather than simple awareness. The first is conceptual reflectivity, which is a kind of bridge between the first four forms and the last three, and where consciousness of awareness, and questioning of the perception that allows this awareness, are present. Psychic reflectivity is the recognition that judgements are made on perceived evidence which may be limited and is certainly influenced by the experiences and awareness of the perceiver. The highest of these three, and therefore of the seven, is what Mezirow describes as the theoretical reflectivity, which is the addition to psychic reflectivity of the capacity to see that although judgements made are limited by personal experience and culture, this is not unchanging, and more useful and satisfying judgements might be made using altered perspectives. This perspective transformation relies on conscious and critical awareness and leads to growth and development of the individual. While it is necessary to separate these seven forms for the purpose of understanding Mezirow's concept, it is perhaps more useful to see them as points on a continuum, with reflectivity as the starting point leading to an infinity of perspective transformation.

This concept is vastly different from Kolb's where action and reflection are antagonists. Mezirow, with his awareness of action at all levels and his juxtaposition of thoughts, perceptions, actions and habits appears to view them as aspects of the whole, rather than as separate in themselves. His use of habit is also interesting in the context of reflectivity. It might be considered that habit opposes reflection, since it leads to routine actions and unthinkingness. By incorporating habit into his levels of reflectivity, the seeker after reflection is forced to consider habits, possibly of long standing, and this consideration may in itself lead to perspective transformation. This linking of action and reflection and the incorporation of habits are also important in Schon's work on reflection-in-action.

Reflection-in-action

Reflection-in-action develops the concept of reflection further, adding the idea of reflecting while acting, rather than post action. Reflection-in-action is more than this, however, and the underlying philosophy is important here. This is based on both Schon's own work and that done in conjunction with Argyris on theory in practice (1974 and 1978). Note that this is not theory related to practice nor theory applied to practice, but theory which is an integral part of practice, and which has grown through the experience of varying practice.

Reflection-in-action is also concerned with the professional relationship, where the professional is seen not as the expert offering solutions to problems, but as someone with particular skills and knowledge who may be able to help a client. The relationship is one of equals, with the client deciding whether or not the professional may be helpful. Within reflection-in-action, Schon has discussed several concepts of use to professionals, including nurses.

The first of these is the idea of theories-in-use. He suggests that the theories-in-use underlying a professional's actions are different from what he refers to as the espoused theories, that is the ones professed to be used. This has been rigorously researched by Schon, both alone (1983) and with Argyris (1974 and 1978). The reasons for this difference are complex, but one of them has to do with the difficulty of relating conventional academic knowledge to actual practice. Schon refers to this conventional academic knowledge as technical rationality, with the basis of this being the formal scientific approach. He is not however saying that this technical rational basis is not useful, rather that it needs to be used in conjunction with knowledge developed from practice, and that this latter type of knowledge may be the more influential.

Reflection-in-action implies awareness of the individual's own theories-in-use. These theories in use, once developed, can be tested in practice and Schon sees reflective practitioners as researchers, although not in the sense of large, conventional research studies, rather as individual action researchers, trying out solutions and using the knowledge gained to assist in future practice.

This view is akin to Kelly's (1963) view of humans as scientists, experimenting on their environment. Kelly is careful to insist that experience in itself does not necessarily make for valid knowledge, that this depends on the validity of the constructs of the person, and that only the reconstruing of events leads to development or learning. Schon does not refer to Kelly in his writings but many of his views reflect similar ideas to those inherent in personal construct theory, developed by Kelly.

A further important concept is the recognition that professional practitioners do not generally deal with the type of problems solvable by reference to technical rational means, rather they encounter very individual, complex, messy and indeterminate situations, demanding an individual and innovative approach. Professionals are taught how to solve problems, but the real problem is how to define the problem from the real-life situation. Problem framing or problem setting is the skill professional practitioners acquire with experience – sometimes.

Schon (1987) states that:

'these indeterminate zones of practice – uncertainty, uniqueness and value conflict – escape the canons of technical rationality. When a problematic solution is uncertain, technical problem solving depends on the prior construction of a well formed problem – which is not itself a technical task.'

Tacit knowledge (Polanyi 1966) is also seen by Schon as a key component in reflection-in-action. 'We know more than we can say' (ibid) is seen as contributing to unique solutions for problems, described by Schon as knowing-in-action. This is linked to Freire's (1972) concept of conscientisation and certainly awareness raising is essential if past experience is to be used to assist present and future practice. The routinisation of practice is called overlearning by Schon, and implies unthinking, unhelpful caregiving, with little possibility of learning from experience.

The other side of this is the use of disjuncture, where learning may occur because something is out of place and does not fit into the common pattern. This disjuncture will cause a fresh view to be taken of the situation and a reframing of the problem. This is similar to Mezirow's (1981) perspective transformation where disjuncture plays a key part. Mezirow's work also stresses the rigour of 'critical reflection' which addresses the validity of taken-for-granted presuppositions' (Mezirow 1988). This examination of assumptions again echoes Schon.

Value conflict is also seen as a major area of concern. Schon discusses the indeterminate areas of practice, where there is no clear-cut solution and where value conflict often exists, unrecognised or unresponded to by the professional practitioner. He relates this to the crisis of confidence in professions generally and states 'that the most important areas of professional practice now lie beyond the conventional boundaries of professional competence' (Schon 1987). Certainly in nursing this is increasingly true and it may be that a move towards professional learning based on the practice exemplar is the way to resolve this. Knowledge developed from practice is relativist and takes account of value conflict, unlike conventional, technical rational knowledge which is positivist and claims to be value free.

IMPLICATIONS FOR NURSING PRACTICE

Nursing practice is continually changing and developing, both because of medical technology and also through wider developments in health care and as a result of social changes. In addition nursing itself is growing through both research and innovative practice, and this may be considered more influential, as well as possibly more important, than the changes brought about by the extrinsic factors.

Certainly nurses are beginning to recognise the satisfaction to be gained from a more in-depth approach to patient problems, and are rejecting routinised practices to a greater extent than a few years ago. The initial education of nurses still concentrates on a narrow foundation of skills, with a somewhat superficial theory base. This is changing with Project 2000 but for any real change to take place, the practice areas must become more valued as areas where nursing practice is the primary source of learning. This is also beginning to be recognised by related professions, most notably social work (Gould 1989).

Mezirow's premise that 'meaning is central to learning'

(Mezirow 1988) is a statement of the obvious in nursing. The difficulties experienced by learner nurses over past decades can be clearly related to the difficulty of finding meaning in being expected to discuss and apply theory taught in the schools of nursing, which is not only not used on the wards, but is frequently denigrated by the clinical staff.

Mezirow's definition of learning is also more useful for professionals and for preparing those for entry to a profession:

'learning may be best understood as the process of construing and appropriating a new or revised interpretation of the meaning of one's experience as a guide to decision and action' (Mezirow 1988).

This concentration on experience and on consciously trying to learn from it, through reflection-in-action, will develop a new practitioner, one who is not only competent immediately following registration, but who in effectiveness grows throughout his or her career. A further development here is the contribution such practitioners will undoubtedly make to nursing knowledge. The critical examination of assumptions, and the alertness to disjuncture, will enable this knowledge to be not mere assertion, but a rigorously examined and valid contribution.

Therapeutic practice, given the dynamic nature of nursing, requires not only a sound foundation of nursing knowledge and skills, but the ability to learn fruitfully throughout the professional career. The suggestion here is that the most useful and appropriate way to achieve this is by using reflective techniques, and by valuing the learning gained from experience.

This may mean substantial changes in attitude by both clinical practitioners and nurse educators. For clinical practitioners, the viewing of practice as a learning experience for themselves and as something to be inculcated in learner nurses, is a major difference, and one which cannot be accomplished by the practitioners without considerable support and assistance in the learning of reflective techniques and their use in therapeutic practice. Should this be achieved, it will not only have a profound effect on learner nurses but on practice itself, enabling it to become more confident and forward thinking, with a willingness to explore and test innovations in practice.

For nurse educators it has even greater implications. The need to be involved in actual practice to a significant extent is evident, but also implied is the need to learn different teaching techniques. These are mainly facilitative, helping learner nurses to evaluate and re-evaluate their experiences. However, the ability to look critically at experience and question taken-for-granted asssumptions needs also to be seen as a priority. This is difficult with the danger of facilitators projecting their own learning experiences and feelings on to the learners, thus undervaluing and undermining the learners' own experiences and making it difficult for them to develop reflecting practice.

Clinical practitioners and nurse educators both need reflective skills and the ability to analyse and evaluate information, whether from formal sources or from experience. The high level of critical skills needed for this is something that few current practitioners or nurse educators possess, although many have the potential, and this will be a major stumbling block in the development of reflective practice. However, nurses have in the past shown great ability to develop and to put major innovations into practice, so these stumbling blocks are not insurmountable. It may be that reflective practice develops slowly but those nurses who aspire to therapeutic practice will recognise the need to learn from experience, and the help that reflective techniques can provide. Possibly in the future, a new epistemology of practice will be the result.

REFERENCES

Argyris, C. and Schon, D. (1974) *Theory in Practice: Increasing Professional Effectiveness*, Addison Wesley, Massachusetts.
Argyris, C. and Schon, D. (1978) *Organisational Learning: A Theory of Action Perspective*, Addison Wesley, Massachusetts.
Benner, P. (1984) *From Novice to Expert, Excellence and Power in Clinical Nursing Practice*, Addison Wesley, California.
Boud, D., Keogh, R. and Walker, D. (eds.) (1985) *Reflection: Turning Experience Into Learning*, Kogan Page, London.
Boud, D. and Griffin, V. (eds.) (1987) *Appreciating Adults Learning*, Kogan Page, London.
Boyd, E.M. and Fales, A.W. (1983) 'Reflective learning: key to learning from experience', *Journal for Humanistic Psychology*, **23** (2), 99–117.
Clarke, M. (1986) 'Action and reflection: practice and theory in

nursing', *Journal of Advanced Nursing*, **11**(1), 3–11.
Dewey, J. (1929) *Experience and Nature*, Grave Press, New York.
Dewey, J. (1933) *How We Think*, D.C. Heath, Boston.
Elliot, J. (1983) 'Self-evaluation, professional development and accountability', Galton, M. and Moon, R., *Changing Schools . . . Changing Curriculum*, 183–201, Kogan Page, London.
Garrison, K. (1964) *Educational Psychology*, Appleton-Century-Crofts, New York.
Garry, R. and Kingsley, H. (1970) *The Nature and Conditions of Learning*, Prentice Hall, New Jersey.
Goldstein, H. (1985) *Social Learning and Change*, Tavistock Publications Ltd., London.
Gould, N. (1989) 'Reflective learning for social work practice', *Social Work Education*, **8**(2), p. 9.
Habermas, J. (1971) *Knowledge and Human Interests*, Beacon Press, Boston.
Harmer, B. and Henderson, V. (1955) *Textbook of the Principles and Practice of Nursing*, Macmillan, New York.
Jarvis, P. and Gibson, S. (1985) *The Teacher Practitioner in Nursing, Midwifery and Health Visiting*, Croom Helm, Beckenham.
Kemmis, S. (1985) 'Action research and the politics of reflection', Boud, D., Keogh, R. and Walker, D. (eds) *Reflection: Turning Experience into Learning*, Kogan Page, London.
Knowles, M.S. (1985) *Andragogy in Action*, Jossey Bass, San Francisco.
Kolb, D.A. (1984) *Experiential Learning*, Prentice Hall, London.
Kolb, D.A. and Fry, R. (1975) 'Towards an applied theory of experiential learning', Cooper, C.L. (ed.) *Theories of Group Processes*, John Wiley & Sons Ltd., London.
Lewin, K. (1935) *A Dynamic Theory of Personality*, McGraw Hill, New York.
Marsick, V. (ed.) (1987) *Learning in the Workplace*, Croom Helm, London.
Mezirow, J. (1981) 'A critical theory of adult learning and education', *Adult Education*, **32**(1), 3–24.
Mezirow, J. (1988) 'Transformation theory', Adult Educators' Conference Paper, South East.
Osborne, A.F. (1953) *Applied Imagination*, Scribners, New York.
Paterson, J. and Zderad, L. (1988) *Humanistic Nursing*, National League for Nursing, New York.
Polanyi, N. (1967) *The Tacit Dimension*, Doubleday and Co. New York.
Procter, S. (1989) 'The functioning of nursing routines in the management of a transient workforce', *Journal of Advanced Nursing*, **14**(3) p. 180.
Schon, D. (1983) *The Reflective Practitioner*, Temple Smith, London.
Schon, D. (1987) *Educating the Reflecting Practitioner*, Jossey Bass, San Francisco.
Shotter, J. (1974) 'What it is to be human', Armistead, R. (ed.), *Reconstructing Social Psychology*, Penguin, Harmondsworth.
Urban, H. and Ford, D. (1971) 'Some historical and conceptual

perspectives on psychotherapy and behaviour change', in Bergin, A. and Garfield, S. (eds) *Handbook of Psychotherapy and Behaviour Change*, John Wiley & Sons Ltd., New York.

Wittgenstein, L. (1974) *Philosophical Investigations*, Trans. Anscombe, G.E.M. Basil Blackwell, Oxford.

Chapter 3

A search for the therapeutic dimensions of nurse–patient interaction

STEVEN ERSSER

This chapter will introduce the issues, method and interim findings of the first stage of fieldwork from an ongoing study designed to explore the views of nurses and patients on how the nursing provided is believed to affect the welfare of patients in hospital.

It is unconventional to view nursing itself as a potential therapy though the nursing literature does make clear reference to the nursing service's objective to foster health. For example, the theoretical writing of nurses over the last century reflect a consensus in the broad purpose of the service to enhance health (Meleis 1985), although few theorists refer directly to the 'therapeutic' dimensions of nursing. Exceptions include Peplau (1952), Travelbee (1966) and Orem (1980). Hockey (1989) has described 'therapeutic nursing' as nursing which leads to health.

A METHOD TO DEVELOP INSIGHTS

This study aims to identify whether hospital nurses and adult patients on medical units hold views about the therapeutic (beneficial) and anti-therapeutic (adverse) effect of nursing and if this is found to be so, to identify the nature of such views and to compare the views of patient and nurse groups. Ultimately, an attempt will be made to develop a conceptual framework from the data. The methodological difficulties involved in studying the therapeutic effect of nursing are now examined and a case is argued for studying this area from the perspective of nurses and patients.

A comlex interplay of factors impinge on the welfare of the hospitalised patient. Nursing is one of the factors likely to affect the patient's health, so there is difficulty identifying the impact of nursing on the patient in isolation from the influence of the social or the physical environment. Furthermore, it could not be assumed that patients or even nurses viewed nursing in itself as a healing activity. Do patients and nurses view nursing as a discrete adjunct or integral part of the medical treatment regimen?

A study of the insider's view; a qualitative research design

A qualitative research design was selected as a suitable design for the study aims. This approach would enable the researcher to document and interpret that which was being studied in particular contexts, from the viewpoint or frame of reference of the people being studied (Leininger 1985). Qualitative research may generate descriptive data on nursing phenomena which are poorly understood. Nursing theory may be derived by deduction from other sciences, however, there is a lack of nursing theory derived inductively from practice, from which researchers may deduce. Qualitative research may be used to develop theory or its component parts which can provide nurses with new insights into the area under study. The concepts and the relationships between them (propositions), from which theory is built, are derived through use of inference by identifying patterns from the study of specific instances (Field and Morse 1985). The product of qualitative research, a theory or its components, also serves as a foundation for further research which tests theory using the hypothetico-deductive method.

Qualitative designs are used when attempting to understand rather than measure phenomena of concern to nurses and allow richly descriptive data to be collected on the meanings situations have for people (Leininger 1985). Social behaviour may be explained on the basis that people will act in accordance with the sense they make of the situation in which they engage (Harrè and Secord 1972). These meanings, arising during social interactions, may influence the outcome of the encounter between nurse and patients.

A qualitative design allows the researcher to draw on the insights gained by nurses on the effect of their actions on patients and on the patient's experience of being nursed. The study of these viewpoints would be of value for several reasons. A fundamental concern of nursing is the attempt to understand and respond to the patient's reaction to their illness, or disability, treatment and care (Wilson-Barnett 1984). In comparison with other health workers, nurses often work in close and frequent contact with patients in helping them to meet needs which they would normally meet themselves. Also, patients are in a position to identify changes in their condition. This experience is important because health is subjectively defined for the individual.

There is no certainty that the views of nurses and patients on the effect of nursing on patients reflect the actual effect endured by patients. However, such views may point to those aspects of nurse-patient interaction requiring further study.

An ethnographic approach

The qualitative approach used in this study is ethnography. The term ethnography also refers to the product of research which is a description and analysis of aspects of the way of life of a particular culture or sub-cultural groups (Germain 1986). In this study the nurse and patient participants constitute sub-cultural groups. Ethnography involves the description of culture, the acquired knowledge of what people use to interpret experience and generate social behaviour (Spradley 1979). People learn their culture by observing other people, listening to them, making inferences from this information. The ethnographer employs the same approach to infer what people know. Culture is a shared system of meanings; a significant part of any culture consists of tacit knowledge. This study made an attempt to identify the knowledge or shared meanings related to the study area and held by the sub-cultural groups under study.

Interactionism and ethnomethodology represent two of the theoretical perspectives which may underlie the ethnographic method. Interactionism is based on the premise that people act on the basis of the meaning a situation has for them and that these meanings arise out of a person's interaction with others (Blumer 1969). Ethnomethodology is based on the premise that social activities have an orderly quality in the way that they are produced by those who participate in them; everyday social activities are seen to have a 'self-organising character' which may be identified (Cuff and Payne 1984). Hammersley and Atkinson (1983) propose an integrated stance to ethnography, arguing that social research is based upon refinements of methods people use in everyday life. The researcher is recognised as part of the world being studied and so rather than attempt to eliminate the observer, the research practices themselves are recognised as a central topic of study (the reflexive principle). An attempt was made in this study to adopt such an approach to ethnography.

Ethnography may be used to identify discrepancies in patient and professional perceptions (Ragucci 1972); it may also contribute to uncovering the complexities of nursing practice and the development of nursing theory (Aamodt 1982), particularly grounded theory (Spradley 1979). Grounded theory or its elements may be discovered during a process of concurrent data collection and analysis. This study aims to identify the logical unity of those concepts and their relationships emerging from the data in an attempt to throw light on the therapeutic dimensions of nursing.

Organisation of the study

The first stage of fieldwork was of three months duration. Three methods were used to collect the data; diaries (document); in-depth ethnographic interviews and group discussions (nurses only). In overview, data collection began with patients completing diaries. These were analysed and used as a basis for drawing up an interview schedule. Two interviews were planned for each participant, to allow for elaboration and clarification of the informants' accounts. The second interview was conducted following the analysis of the first. The study was organised with the aim that nurses on the same ward remain unaware of the content of the diary and interview process for the patient participants. Data collection involving the patient was followed by that for the nurses so as to minimise the nurses' awareness that their actions were being reflected upon while the patients completed their diaries. Therefore it will not be possible to make detailed comparisons of the perspectives of particular nurses and patients during interaction. Nurses commenced with the same pattern of participation as the patients except that they engaged in a group discussion prior to completing their diary.

The setting and sampling methods

The study was set in general and specialty (neurological) medical wards in two different acute hospitals within the same health authority. Nurse and patient participants were selected from these settings. The unit of analysis was the cultural knowledge of hospital nurses and patients on the effect nursing is believed to have on patients. A small number of cases are studied in ethnography (Hammersley and Atkinson 1983). However, these cases were not treated as 'case studies' in which particular individuals are studied in a comprehensive way (Hakim 1987).

The samplng methods were theoretically directed with informants being selected who would facilitate the development of the emerging theory – described as purposive sampling (Field and Morse 1985). People who had some experience of being nursed were selected, and so patients who had been on the ward for less than one day were excluded. For the first stage of fieldwork the aim was to have included four nurses and four patients as participants whose views on the study area were explored in depth. Due to the deterioration in the condition of one participation and the problems of writing difficulty and lethargy for others only two patients participated at this stage. A greater number of participants will be involved in the second stage of fieldwork. The charge nurse was asked to decide on the fitness of patients to participate. Patients who had not been resident in the UK for at least ten years, and who could not write or speak English, were excluded. The 'nurse' participants included any qualified nurse, student or care assistant who nursed patients. It could not be assumed prior to fieldwork that the different staff grades would hold differing views nor that patients would necessarily observe any differences in their behaviour.

There was also a practical requirement to select accessible informants through opportunistic sampling (Burgess 1984), which was anticipated. This was due to the difficulty selecting patients who were hospitalised for sufficient time for diary recording, interview participation and concurrent data analysis. Furthermore, some patients had difficulty keeping a diary mainly becauses of physical difficulty writing and lethargy. The extent of this problem was not anticipated.

Sampling within the case was also used. It was made clear to the informants that the diary entries could be written in at any time they chose as significant. For the nurse group, those nurses working on night and day shift were invited to participate. Also different types of informant were sought, for example, male and female, older and younger people and nurses of various grades. However, it was not known prior to fieldwork if these variables would be a significant influence on the type of accounts provided.

The development of grounded theory relies on the selection of cases which generate through analysis as many categories from the data as possible (Glaser and Strauss 1967). A form of purposive sampling termed theoretical sampling would be used in which the direction of data collection is guided by the product of ongoing data analysis. It was intended that the use of both a general medical ward (heterogeneous patient group) and a specialty medical ward (homogeneous) could also serve as cases for comparison.

Data collection methods

The diaries consisted of unstructured notebooks with an accompanying instruction sheet. They constitute a form of personal documentary data which were completed solely for research purposes. Diaries have been used in social research by Burgess (1983), for example. They were intended to enable the informants to provide spontaneous, personalised accounts, freely structured by them. Informants were asked to consider the following statements, worded as follows for patients:

> 'I am interested in your experiences of receiving nursing care. In particular I want you to try and describe how you believe the nursing you receive affects you.'

The nurse group considered the following:

> 'I am interested in your experiences of giving nursing care.

In particular I want you to try and describe how you believe the nursing you give affects your patients.'

Informants were requested to reflect on this issue and complete the diary as they felt appropriate over a period of up to five days. The ethnographic interviews were intended to serve as a basis for exploring informants' diary entries through allowing the opportunity to request elaboration and clarification. Such interviews are said to share many of the features of friendly conversations because they have an informal quality (Burgess 1984). The interview schedules served as flexible *aide-mémoires* in providing a list of topics and questions.

'Ethnographic elements' were introduced during the interview including explanations about its purpose and the use of ethnographic questions (Spradley 1979). Descriptive questions were used to get informants to talk about aspects of the cultural scene, for example, the nurses may be asked 'What is it like working as a nurse on this ward?' Structural questions were used to identify the basic units of the informants' cultural knowledge related to the study aims. Informants were often asked to give more information about the behaviour of nurses or its affect on the patient referred to in the diary. The different meanings of words expressed by the informants would be distinguished using contrast questions. For example 'You have referred to the nurse's ''friendly gestures'' and ''friendly manner''; did you see these as the same or different in some way?' Ethnographic interviews also involve the expression of cultural ignorance by the ethnographer who may ask 'What did you mean by the word ''relationship''?' or 'Could you explain to me what ''doing the obs'' involves?' As a nurse it is important that the ethnographer does not take the meanings underlying language for granted. Interviews were tape recorded to provide an accurate record and to avoid note-taking during conversation.

The group discussions involved the two nurse participants, and one or two nurses who were not participating from the same ward who were free to leave the ward and the ethnographer. This method has been used in other studies such as that of Stimpson and Webb (1975). Group discussions were intended only for use with the nurse participants for several reasons. Diary completion requires a commitment from nurses which may be difficult to keep while working; an opportunity was needed to discuss this. Two potential problems were envisaged: that nurses may have difficulty recording the adverse effects of their action and may become overwhelmed by the broad nature of the diary question, since they had been socialised into coming to know the numerous ways in which they may affect patients. Through acknowledging that these concerns may arise it was hoped that keeping a diary would become less problematic. In practice, the nurse participants had few difficulties despite initial apprehension. The opportunity for dialogue on the diary question also allowed different perspectives on the diary question to be identified. Furthermore, the discussions were intended to help nurses to focus on the exercise and to provide a basis to explore the use of 'public' and 'private' accounts. The format of the group discussion was informal and semi-structured using the agenda described above. Explanations about the study were given, the diary question was discussed and the practicalities and potential difficulties of keeping a diary raised.

Methodological notes were kept by the ethnographer in a fieldwork journal immediately after any involvement in the fieldwork setting. These are the personal reflections on the ethnographer's field activities such as access and adaptation of the methods used (Burgess 1984). This process was necessary since the ethnography was recognised as a part of the social world being studied.

Analysis of data: content analysis
and constant comparative method

Diaries and interviews were transcribed verbatim to provide accurate and detailed records. The diary transcripts and tape recordings of interviews and group discussions were treated as the primary data source. Data analysis took place during the fieldwork period allowing further data collection to be guided in the form of theoretical sampling.

To develop 'grounded theory' it was first necessary to identify categories within the data. Categories are conceptual elements of the emerging theory and were identified using content analysis; this involves classifying the contents of communication so as to bring out their basic structure (Abercrombie et al. 1988). Analysis began with the identification and labelling of units of meaning within the data through a process of coding (Corbin 1986). Germain (1986) said that the cultural inferences drawn by the ethnographer are the scientists' meaning of the meanings communicated by the informants. For this study the units of meaning encompassed any expressions of belief in the existence of a relationship between the behaviour of the nurse(s) and its effect on the patient and an account of the context in which this took place. Coding involved searching out these three elements and labelling the code (a conceptual label) according to the behaviour of the nurse.

For each code developed a brief theoretical note was made to explain thoughts while coding. Following the coding of the first transcript memos were then written to capture the recurring ideas observed in the data (Corbin 1986). Memos are the write up of theoretical ideas about codes and their relationships (Glaser 1978). A memo fund was developed and sorted as data came in. The memos served to guide the analysis by providing a record of what had been identified and where the direction of further data collection should go. Different types of memos were written at the different stages of analysis. Category memos were to be developed to discover categories. Comparative memos were used to build categories through identifying their characteristics (Glaser 1978); the similarities and differences between codes and the different cases under study (patients, nurses and wards) would be explored. This process is integral to the development of grounded theory. In order to link the categories further memos would be written to explore hypotheses about the relationship between categories. Due to the limited amount of data available by the end of the first stage of fieldwork it was only possible to begin to write such memos once the initial coding of data from the second stage of fieldwork was complete.

During the next stage of analysis the aim is to develop the general design or conceptual framework which represents the major pattern of organisation of the area of social life under study (Lofland 1971); this phase of analysis is at its early stages as more second stage fieldwork data is being analysed. Memos are being written to integrate previous memos into an account which aimed at identifying the central idea of the phenomenon under study. Also diagrams are being drawn up which provide a visual representation of the analytic scheme to help explore the links between categories (Corbin 1986).

The data now presented is derived from the first stage of fieldwork. As such it can only illuminate some of the areas of interest at an arbitrary interim stage of analysis. However, initial coding of the second stage fieldwork data indicates that the three major dimensions of the data introduced below continue to emerge as such.

The existence of views about the therapeutic effect of nursing

Various sets of data will be used to illustrate the informants' identification of a relationship existing between specific behaviour of a nurse (or nurses) and the patient's welfare. For brevity the sets are sometimes confined to a description of the nurses' behaviour only. These data sets are labelled according to their source; transcripts are coded 'D' for diary and 'I' for interview. The number before the colon refers to the interview number and that after the colon to the page number.

Ethnography involves open-ended inquiry in which the ethnographer's initial aims may be altered by discoveries made during fieldwork. As such it could not be assumed prior to fieldwork that nurses and patients may hold views on how nurses were believed to affect patients. From the first-stage fieldwork it was evident that nurse and patient participants held views on the effect of nursing on patients. For example:

1. Nurse A (D: 6)   *'I spent as much time as possible (today) helping her to drink'*

   'D, who has a stroke, is having great difficulty drinking so I spent as much time as possible today helping her to drink so that hopefully she will not have to go back on I.V.I. hydration which is both uncomfortable and an infection risk.'

From the data it is evident that the nurse and patient participants typically did not make specific reference to the effect of nursing on the patient's 'health'. The effect was described in more general terms as having beneficial or adverse consequences for the patient. For example:

2. Nurse F (I1: 18)   *A listening ear*

'There were several people who may have had bad news after investigations, like cancer – a cancerous growth or something, and they, I think, were thinking about that in their head, although you never can tell . . . so to listen to them would do them quite a lot of good, I think, well, in general it does anyway.'

Further illustrations of both nurse's and patient's views exist throughout the chapter.

THE NATURE OF NURSES' AND PATIENT VIEWS

From 19 transcripts of nurses and patients obtained so far 13 themes (groups of related categories) and 30 categories of the themes have emerged. The themes are clusters of related categories and as such represent broader categories of the conceptual elements of the emerging theory. Themes and categories are formed from the codes described earlier and as such are also labelled according to the nurse's behaviour described. Even larger units of meaning which encompass

Table 3.1 Units of data obtained through content analysis: an example from nurses' accounts

Dimension	Theme	Category	Property
Presentation	The Nurse	Nurse feeling tired and/or not in the mood	[Problems arising from mood/tiredness]
			Difficulty being receptive/sensitive to patients.
			Avoiding contact with patient
			Being busy and feeling overtired
			Difficulty giving explanation (also, due to lack of time)

and extend across the themes were identified; these were termed 'dimensions'. Examples are given in Table 3.1.

Dimensions emerging from first stage fieldwork (FSF)

From the content analysis of the data from the first stage of fieldwork three dimensions have emerged. It is interesting that the same three dimensions have been identified in *both* the nurses' and patients' data. Each dimension describes a facet of the nurse's (or group of nurses) behaviour which is believed by the informants to produce a beneficial or adverse effect in the patient.

Table 3.2 Dimensions of first stage fieldwork

Dimension	*Views placing emphasis on:*
1) The presentation of the nurse	– How the nurse appears before the patient (Largely non-verbal behaviour)
2) The presence of the nurse	– The nurse proximity to the patient or 'being with' the patient
3) The specific actions of the nurse	– The specific-procedural-type activities of the nurse

Only the first phase of data analysis on the data derived from the second six month stage of fieldwork has been conducted so far. However, it is evident that the three dimensions as described above continue to emerge.

EXPLORING VIEWS ABOUT THE THERAPEUTIC EFFECT OF NURSE-PATIENT INTERACTION

Travelbee (1971) describes 'nurse-patient interaction' as any contact between a nurse and an ill person and 'relationships' as an experience or series of experiences which are mutually significant. Numerous references have been made in the literature to the potential therapeutic qualities of the nurse-patient relationship (such as Peplau 1952; and Muetzal 1988). The therapeutic features of staff-client relationships are commonly described in the field of psychiatry (such as Altschul 1972, and see section on 'therapeutic use of self'). The therapeutic effect of relationships are the subject of research in social psychology (Duck 1984) but this remains at an early stage of development.

To identify if the features of interaction referred to in the participants' accounts of this study are of the type described as a 'relationship' it is necessary to explore the concept further. A 'relationship' is a difficult entity to define (Altschul 1972). Argyle and Henderson (1985) have described a 'relationship' as '. . . regular social encounters with certain people over a period of time . . . together with the expectation that this will continue for at least some time into the future'. It is difficult to assess from the data if the experiences between the nurses and patients involved are 'mutually significant', however, it is possible that some of them may be, and furthermore, it appears that many of the experiences recalled in the accounts occur as regular social encounters. As such, it seems reasonable to assume that some of the features of interaction, such as 'presence' or 'presentation', may represent facets of a 'relationship' existing between nurse and patient. From the current data the features of nurse-patient interaction which are viewed by the participants as beneficial infrequently make explicit reference to a 'relationship'. It may be that dimensions of interaction identified in this study may exist irrespective of whether a relationship has been formed. Alternatively, the existence of a nurse-patient relationship may be implicit in the participants' accounts because it is taken for granted.

The remaining focus of the chapter will be confined to the dimensions of the data which are less frequently referred to in the nursing literature, 'presentation' and 'presence'.

THE PRESENTATION OF THE NURSE

Data obtained so far reveal that both nurse and patient believe that the way the nurse presents herself in the presence of the patient may have a bearing on the patient's well-being. This takes various forms including the nurse's attitude and manner, the nurse's appearance and whether behaviour conveys confidence.

The most salient theme in the data of both nurses and

patients, in terms of the range and frequency of views expressed, were those encompassed by the theme 'the nurse'. This includes sets of views referring to the personal qualities of the nurse which are believed to be important influences on the outcome of interaction with the patient. This theme will be used to illustrate the dimension of 'presentation' using the following sections of data (data sets). Due to the 'rich' nature of the data emerging, and the large range of views expressed, only a very limited number of data sets may be described.

3. Nurse W (D: 8)   '. . . *my attitude to my work, my patients and the care I give'*

'I can make a patient feel welcome, or at ease, or not. I can make them feel I am dictating care, giving care, neglecting care, encouraging self-care-involvement, preventive care and awareness all by my approach and attitude.'

4. Patient L (D: 1)   '*A friendly manner'*

'The nurses are often the only people I get to chat to and being treated in a friendly manner helps to alleviate loneliness. . .'

5. Patient L (I1: 39)   '*Nervous nurses'*
   [Nurse looking after a patient with a tracheostomy who needs to learn to manage it herself]

'. . . I would've felt happier about the whole thing if people had been more confident – I mean, when you get a nurse come in and she's too frightened to clean it, it doesn't exactly make you feel sort of confident with it.'

Both nurse and patient participants refer to the significance of non-verbal aspects of the nurses' behaviour, such as facial expression or nervous demeanour, and the emotional effect this may have on the patient, however transient. An example from a nurse participant is given below. There is also some indication' from the patient group of a belief on how the nurse's presentation may influence the effectiveness of their subsequent interaction with the nurse.

6. Nurse F (I1: 46)   *'Difficulty being receptive/sensitive to patient's needs due to nurse feeling "overtired" or not in the "mood"'*

'. . . perhaps just an odd tut, or your facial expression, mine particularly – I know, change according to my mood and not necessarily a smiling face! You may not meet their physical and emotional needs.'

Patient accounts reflected two categories within this theme not referred to by nurses: 'Having confidence or not in the nurse to meet expectations' and the 'Nurse with a sense of humour' (below).

7. Patient L (D: 4)   *Nurse with a sense of humour*

'10.30 p.m. finally got my trachy cleaned. The nurse said she'd only ever cleaned one before years ago. Wouldn't it be nice to have someone who knew what they were doing? She asked me what to do . . . she had a good sense of humour and treated me like a normal person so it didn't matter so much that she wasn't used to doing them.'

8. Patient L (D: 7)   *Having confidence in the nurse to know what they are doing*

'. . . I appreciate the nurses being friendly and it's great when they have time to chat but it would be beneficial to have confidence in them and this has been difficult because they are not familiar with the treatment of tracheotomies.'

A sociological analysis of 'Presentation of the Nurse'

'Information about the individual helps to define the situation, enabling others to know how best to act in order to call forth a desired response from him' Goffman (1971, p. 13).

A sociological perspective will be used to illuminate the significance of this dimension. Earlier, reference was made to the premises of the theoretical perspective of interactionism that the behaviour of people in a situation is related to the meaning that the situation has for them. An understanding of action in nursing therefore requires an interpretation of the meanings which nurses and patients give to nurses' actions. For example, the patient 'L' defines the situation above differently from that described in (7) because the nurse's actions have a different meaning for her. In consequence the patient modifies her expectations of the nurse and the distress experienced previously is not reported.

The manner in which the nurse and patient define their situation will shape the way they will act subsequently. Their actions will depend on the interpretation of the behaviour of each party by the other. This process of 'making sense' takes place during interaction and involves negotiation. Each party will attempt to acquire information about the other. Mutual expectations will be held about how the other party will act. Viewed in this way the presentation of the nurse may influence the outcome of nursing care for the patient. For example, the patient's distress described in data set 9 is shown to be minimised by the nurse's sense of humour (set 7).

9. Patient L (D: 1)   *'Conflicting advice' (a specific action of the nurse)*

'People constantly have different ideas about care . . . This has caused me a lot of distress – it's unnerving to be told different things.'

This example shows that despite the same display of technical incompetence in the specific action of the nurse and lack of awareness of the patient's needs, the nurse 'presentation' in the form of an expression of humour, is believed by the patient (data set 7) to influence the outcome of the encounter differently from the experience recalled in data set 9.

The relationship of the presentation of the nurse to patient outcome is depicted in Figure 3.1.

PRESENTATION DEFINITION OF   MUTUAL   ACTION OF
OF NURSE - - - SITUATION - - - EXPECTATIONS - - - - - EACH PARTY
              (MAKING SENSE) (about desirability
                              of each party's actions)
                                                    may influence
                                                    PATIENT OUTCOME

Figure 3.1 A sociological analysis of the presentation of the nurse and its relationship to patient outcome.

The social meaning of the nurse's emotional display and its consequences for the patient

Social acts convey meaning and this applies to the actions of the nurse. An illustration is provided by Chapman (1983) in a study of rituals in hospitals. The frequent references to the emotional expression of the nurse in the accounts so far suggests that such behaviour may be an important influence on the construction of meanings in nurse-patient interaction. The accounts related to the 'presentation of the nurse' include reference to the nurse's emotional behaviour. The outward appearance of a nurse's emotions are viewed as having the potential to affect the patient. The term 'emotional display' will be used to refer to such expressions of emotion. Weber was concerned with the meaning and intention behind social behaviour (Roth and Wittch 1978). He viewed 'affectual (emotional) action' as unintentional and not purposefully directed in a rational way since it is defined as distinct from 'rational action'. However, the accounts presented here encompass both intentional action (emotions which have been 'worked on' by the nurse) and 'natural' unintentional expressions of affect which are truly felt.

Emotional labour and intentional emotional display

'. . . I assume that when an individual appears before others he will have many motives for trying to control the impression they receive of the situation.' Goffman (1971)

The deliberate management of emotional appearance in social interaction for instrumental purposes is described by Hochschild (1983) in her book *The Managed Heart: the Commercialisation of Human Feeling*. In a study of air hostesses she introduces the concept of 'emotional labour' (7) as:

'. . . the management of feeling to create a publically observable facial or bodily display: emotional labour is sold for a wage and therefore has exchange value.'

Hochschild viewed emotional labour as a form of social engineering within public service work believing that the emotional work of women is used to affirm, enhance and celebrate the well-being and status of others. Her work draws on empirical examples using observation and interview from a range of sources. Smith's work (1988) identified that nurses were engaging in emotional labour by being requested to produce an emotional state in another, such as gratitude, and having face-to-face contact with the public.

There is further evidence in the study presented here of the capacity of nurses' deliberate use of their emotions to influence the patient's welfare. This is illustrated in data set 3. It is difficult, however, to identify whether the emotional display of the nurse is deliberate in the sense of being 'managed' or not.

In making sense of each interaction the patient may make judgements about the sincerity of the nurses' actions. Although many of the patient accounts so far do not highlight this point, (such as data set 4) there are indications of such awareness, for example:

10. Patient E (D: 1–2)   *A kind genuine smile*

'. . . as a patient one perhaps tends to be perhaps over-sensitive to what seems unkind treatment, whereas a kind genuine smile from anyone does wonders for the patient.'

Jourard (1971) refers to the problems of the 'bedside manner', '. . . a peculiar kind of inauthentic behaviour adopted by nurses.' (177)

Different forms of emotional display have been described in the literature. Hochschild draws on Goffman's dramaturgical analysis of interactions referring to 'surface acting' and 'deep acting'. 'Surface acting' describes behaviour in which there is a change in the outward appearance of a person with the action being in the body language. It is a way of deliberately disguising what is really being felt, there is no self deception. 'Deep acting', however, involves a display which results naturally from working on feeling; the person tries to feel what they believe they ought or want to feel through the production of real self-induced feelings in a way often used by actors.

Belief in the use of surface acting by nurses is to some extent evident in both nurses' and patients' accounts, but, it is not always easy to define them as referring to one type or another. This is exemplified in data set 3. The cases of emotional display described could involve either surface acting or unintentional displays because the nurse or patient does not refer to the nurses's intent in as such, or often assume that it is not anything other than genuine felt emotion (see data sets 5 and 15). The following account reveals a student's growing awareness of her ability to surface act.

11. Nurse A (I1: 37)

'. . . as a nurse you can't sort of totally throw off your mood and be all smiles and chit chat to the patient always. I think, most of the time you can – I'm amazed at myself – how lousy I can feel and yet how, you know, sort of bubbly I can appear sometimes.'

Hochschild selected the extreme case of the airline flight hostess to highlight emotion work in public life and the extent to which emotional labour can go. It appears from the nurses' accounts here that emotional display does not necessarily involve emotion management. Furthermore, the pattern of emotional labour is different from that adopted by flight attendants who would attempt to use a high degree of both surface and deep acting relative to the level of natural display. The context of care services rather than that of the commercial field may largely account for this because the natural expression of interest and concern for another would be more likely to arise in the care context. Furthermore, the high level of stress which often pervades clinical situations may lead to nurse's controlling their own true feelings where possible because of a fear (or perhaps a myth) that such disclosures may threaten their ability to interact successfully with patients.

Natural-unintentional emotional display

The emotional display of the nurse would often appear to involve spontaneous natural expressions which do not constitute emotional labour. Evidence of the genuine expression of emotions was provided in data sets 7 and 9. It is also implicit in this example:

12. Patient L (I1: 12b) *Being friendly 'in a kind of ordinary friendly way'*

'. . . hospital can be a very lonely place – you know I think if you sort of find one or two nurses who are friendly – in a kind of ordinary friendly way – you know what I mean, not just a nurse being friendly but, but just another person being friendly to you – I think that sort of makes me feel less isolated.

Several accounts describe the breakdown of emotional management. In the account below (13) the nurse describes her concern about disclosing her emotions to the patient (see also data set 6).

13. Nurse A (I1: 36)   *Avoiding contact*

'The thing about standing at the end of the bed hiding behind the charts, that's more to do with how I'm feeling myself. If I do that then it's probably cos I'm not feeling confident. But, just sometimes you don't feel like it, you're just not in the mood to sort of say who you are and what you're there to do . . . I always feel later when I go back to the person, I'm aware that we haven't yet been introduced and it – it would've been easier to have broken the ice earlier.'

The consequences of nurses' emotional display for the patient

The above accounts reflect a belief in the capacity of emotional display to enhance or impair the well-being of the patient. This may be directly or indirectly through influencing the conditions whereby needs may or may not be met.

14. Nurse W (D: 2)   *I try and be friendly and open*

Obviously my attitude when giving out drugs can alter, affect the patient's attitude to myself and nurses in general. If I try to be friendly, open and converse this naturally puts people more at ease, more relaxed.

This account reflects a nurse's conscious awareness of his actions: it is a purposefully directed act with a belief in some degree of cause and effect.

In the patients data the sub-category 'being friendly' of 'the nurse' theme illustrates the patient's belief in the benefit gained from the nurse's friendliness.

15. Patient L (D: 1)   *A friendly manner*

> The nurses are often the only people I get to chat to and being treated in a friendly manner helps to alleviate loneliness.

This was a significant statement when considered in context. This patient had a serious illness on admission and was separated from her husband, who is disabled; furthermore, all her family lived at a great distance from hospital. The sincerity of the nurses' act does not seem in question here. The 'bedside manner' does not appear to be at play. Concern has been expressed that the bedside manner may lead to a neglect of personal needs and feelings of the nurse and serve as an obstacle to communication with the patient, acting specifically as a barrier to a self disclosure (Jourard 1971). However, Jourard recognises the 'armoury function' of the bedside manner, which allows the nurse to work unaffected by excess emotion and insecurity.

During fieldwork Strauss et al. (1982) identified the 'sentimental' work which accompanied instrumental work in hospitals. Several types were described which correspond with the findings emerging from this study. 'Composure work', which may involve an empathic display by the nurse, was found to be the most usual and visible type of sentimental work. It is said to help patients to remain composed during a frightening and/or painful procedure. 'Trust work' depicts the display of many subtle gestures which reflect concern and competence; this may help staff to carry out other work such as an unavoidable painful procedure. Obtaining details about the patient's personal history and life-style ('Biographical work'), like 'Trust work', may help the nurse and patient to relate. The significance of sentimental work is captured by Strauss et al. (1982):

> . . . when the sentimental work is not done, or is done badly in someone's judgement, then not only the main line of medical work may be affected but so may interactions, moods, composures, identities. Patients' feelings of humiliation, insult, invaded privacy, physical and mental discomfort, and resentment at being treated like an object are related to failures of sentimental work.'

Gow (1982) conducted a study on 'How Nurses' Emotions Affect Patient Care'. He studied accounts of situations by 275 graduate nurses in which they believed they were 'helpful' and 'unhelpful' to patients. They were required to identify how they themselves felt prior to and simultaneous with their outward actions in nurse-patient interaction.

The nurses believed their emotions had a significant impact on whether situations were helpful or unhelpful, however they were found to question their motives and skills to nurse people. Nurses believed they were unhelpful to patients due to their self image being threatened; purposefully disregarding significant cues in patients' behaviour and feeling inadequate to address a patient's problem because they themselves had not resolved the issue. They believed that they were constrained by organisational factors such as having too little time to devote to patients. The importance of the time factor is discussed further in the section on the 'presence' of the nurse.

Three main helping responses of the nurse were identified. First, 'gave moral support', which was characterised by the nurse providing verbal reassurance. Second, 'was a sounding board' involved the nurse listening to the patient and thirdly, 'took time to explain'. The following conclusion by Gow (1982) supports the current findings that:

> 'In situations where the nurses saw themselves as helpful, it was not because they perceived that they had neutralised their affect but rather because they had directed their affect in a particular way.'

There is one obvious weakness of method in Gow's work. She made a priori assumptions, in what was intended as an open-ended inquiry, about the capacity of the nurse herself to affect the patient. Gow stated to the participants that the evaluation of the descriptions will be based on '. . . your ability to examine your use of self in each (situation)'.

The 'therapeutic use of self' concept re-examined

The dimension of the data the 'presentation of the nurse' provides an indication from the existing case studies that nurses and patients may hold beliefs about the potential of such behaviour to affect the patient, whether intentional or not. Goffman's concept of the 'presentation of self' places emphasis on the deliberate management of appearances and so it does not, therefore, adequately account for the data on the nurse's emotional display. A similar situation is found with accounts of the concept of the 'therapeutic use of self' described in the literature. Travelbee (1971) defines this as follows:

'When a nurse uses self therapeutically she consciously makes use of her personality and knowledge in order to effect a change in the ill person. This change is considered therapeutic when it alleviates the individual's stress.'

This concept of 'therapeutic use of self' would only account for those features of nurses' emotional display which involve emotional labour and the use of intent. Therefore, there are indications that this concept requires further empirical and theoretical analysis.

The concept of the 'therapeutic use of self'

The concept of the 'therapeutic use of self' has its origins in psychotherapy which is defined by Taylor (1982) as

'Any procedure that promotes the development of courage, inner security and self confidence can be called psychotherapy. However, the traditional use of this term is limited to sustained interpersonal interactions between the psychotherapist and client where the goal is to help the client to develop behaviours that are more functional.'

Reference to the influence of psychotherapy on the theoretical thinking in nursing is evident in the work of Peplau (1952), Travelbee (1971) and Hall (1969). The therapeutic use of self is said to require that the educated heart and the educated mind are used together (Travelbee). The emphasis on the value of the nurse's intentional or purposeful action for the patient is, to some degree, in contrast to the interim findings from the study presented here; these accounts also convey a belief in the potential value of nurse's natural unintentional emotional display for patients.

Peplau (1952) made no direct reference to the term 'therapeutic use of self' but referred to nursing as '. . . an interpersonal process and often a therapeutic one'. Peplau's interest lies in 'psychodyhamic nursing' which she describes as understanding one's own behaviour in order to help others. Like Travelbee, Peplau was concerned with the nurse-patient relationship and its implications for patient welfare.

Balint's (1964) review of psychotherapeutic activity in GP clinics identified that by far the most frequently used 'drug' was the doctor himself. Descriptions tended not to include reference to the emotional display of the doctor but rather specific actions such as the use of understanding and listening (referred to later).

Specific reference to the psychotherapeutic action of the nurse has been made by June Mellow (1966). She used the term 'Nursing Therapy' to refer to '. . . a treatment approach to emotional illness incorporating techniques which range from the nursing process to those used in psychologically orientated psychotherapy'. In this description the role of the nurse is not clearly distinguished from that of the psychotherapist. However, Mellow (like Hall 1969) states her belief in the strategic advantages for the nurse of the opportunities to develop emotional closeness through providing intimate physical care saying that 'Individual therapy is not viewed as something separate and apart from the patient's everyday experiences'. This is a complex issue because the effective use of such opportunities in a way that, at the very least, does not do more harm than good requires tremendous skill on the part of nurses. The issue of the psychotherapeutic role of the nurse has been the subject of debate in the field of psychiatry, particularly in areas such as the therapeutic community (see Weddell 1968, for example). Chapman (1986) would appear sympathetic to some aspects of Mellow's position:

> 'It is the multidimensional aspect of the nurse's role, the requirement that he or she respond appropriately to the varying dimensions of human experience, which separates the nurse's task from that of the psychoanalyst. I would suggest that the nurse mediates between the physiological, psychological, and social experience of patients through action as well as talk.'

It has been said there is a need for nurses in the general field to incorporate concepts from psychotherapy into current practice (Schwartz and Schwartz 1972). However, the complexity of this issue has been rarely addresed. Peplau and Travelbee intended that their ideas would be applied beyond the psychiatric field. Muetzal (1988) and Ersser (1988) describe attempts to explore practice in the field of general nursing working from the premises set out by Hall (1969). Such practices require rigorous study and evaluation in the clinical setting. The study by Pearson et al. (1988) was an attempt to evaluate the effectiveness of nursing beds, based on Hall's premises about nursing as a therapy. However, the evaluation did not extend to the examination of practices such as the non-directive style of nursing in which patients were encouraged to become active participants, when appropriate.

Uys's (1980) descriptive paper attempts to formulate an operational definition of the therapeutic use of self concept. She derived three antecedent steps which were: self knowledge, self growth and scientific knowledge. However, it is interesting that Uys recognises that this does not mean that person cannot have a therapeutic effect within interaction without having gone through the antecedent areas; attributing this capacity either to natural inclination, luck or developed social skill. This point is implicit in the accounts of the study presented here and is one not often expressed in the nursing literature.

PRESENCE

Be near me when I fade away,
To point the term of human strife,
And on the low dark verge of life
The twilight of eternal day.

Be near me when my light is low,
When the blood creeps, and the nerves prick
And tingle; and the heart is sick,
And all the wheels of being slow.

Alfred, Lord Tennyson
'Be near me when the sensuous frame'
in Benn (1986)
With kind permission from Ravette Ltd

The importance of the quality of 'presence' during nurse-patient interaction is evident from the accounts of both parties.

This dimension of the data reflects a belief in the value of the nurse 'being with' or having proximity to the patient, in physical and, or, existential terms. The themes within this dimension are set out in Table 3.3.

Table 3.3 Themes within the dimension of presence: first-stage fieldwork

Nurse Data	Patient Data
1) Making contact with the patient	1) Caring
2) Support and Caring	2) Availability of the nurse
3) Availability of the nurse	3) The Nurse (category 'To
4) The Nurse (category 'Sensitivity/ insensitivity shown to the patient.)	determine what the problem is from the patient's point of view.

A wide range of literature refers to the importance of presence in helping situations; however, few attempts have been made to review and synthesise it. The data provides a framework within which to consider the related literature. The relevant themes are now considered.

Presence as 'making contact with patients'

This theme encompasses views of nurses only and refers to three categories: the nurse initiating, maintaining and avoiding contact with the patient. The accounts convey that the manner in which encounters are initiated, sustained and evaded all have implications for the nurse in her capacity effectively to help the patient. Some of the accounts in the theme 'making contact with patients' are closely related to those accounts within the theme 'availability of the nurse' (such as data set 16). At present they are distinguished by the former theme incorporating references to some of the forms which nurse-patient interaction may take while the latter refers to the nurse's accessibility as construed by nurse or patient.

The nurse's 'presence' with the patient through initiating contact is captured in the following account. Frequent reference is made to the indirect value of presence described in the accounts as a means to create the conditions by which some of the patient's needs may be met.

16. Nurse A (I1: 25)   *Introducing oneself to the patient*

'. . . if you go straight over, sit on their bed and say, ''I'm A and I'll be looking after you this afternoon, is there anything you need now?'' And maybe tell them what you might be doing to them this afternoon, or, whatever, then when you approach them again, they know what you're doing and they will hopefully feel if they do need something they can ask.'

The significance of the opening interaction is also a consequence of the way in which the nurse's 'presentation' contributes to the patient's definition of the situation. The manner in which the nurse initiates contact with the patient is known to be important in helping to alleviate the high anxiety often associated with hospital admission (Wilson-Barnett and Carrigy 1978). 'Maintaining contact' reflects views of the nurse on how the patient may benefit from continuing contact with the nurse. This allows the patient the opportunity to develop trust in the nurse as a basis for forming a relationship. In the following example the relationship is not only viewed as a basis for communication but relating is seen as valuable in its own right.

17. Nurse A (D: 1–2)   *Making contact with patients – a basis for building a comfortable relationship*

'Certainly as a first warder who can't do an awful lot of the more technical things and isn't expected to undertake any management of the ward – I think I do get more contact with the patients. Through this contact if I can build up a relationship with a patient whereby they feel comfortable with me and able to discuss or just tell their worries, problems or share good news, then that is a very positive thing I am doing.'

Reference to the literature on the therapeutic potential of the nurse-patient relationship has been mentioned earlier. No further reference will be made here because the focus of this chapter is on those areas of nurse-patient interaction which are highlighted by the data.

The nurse's frequent contact with the patient was also seen as a means of reducing the patient's feelings of isolation. The following account describes the anxiety of a woman who was immobile due to a neurological disorder. To minimise this patient's anxiety and fear that the nurse may not return the nurse promises to maintain contact.

18. Nurse Sa (I1: 17)   *Endeavouring to make contact with a patient who is to a degree helpless in some way.*

'She was actually having that contact. I think she was very afraid that she couldn't do things for herself, all right . . . she was almost stranded and so we had this thing that we would definitely come back to 'J' to move her legs.'

The category 'avoiding contact' describes the way in which the nurse's avoidance of contact with patients can prevent certain needs being met (see data set 13). Stockwell's (1972) small study found that, almost without exception, nurse-patient interaction was task-initiated and there were observable differences in the ways in which nurses interacted with the most and least popular patients. From the data (set 13) the missed opportunities to develop rapport are evident.

Presence as 'support and caring'

The value of providing patients with 'support' is evident in the nurses' accounts. However, both nurses and patients refer to the importance of 'caring'. Currently the nurse data cannot be clearly differentiated as 'caring' or 'support' because the categories and their characteristics emerging from analysis are not confined to one of these activities. Nurse and patient participants describe caring or support as 'presence' and as being of benefit to the patient. The relevant categories are set out in Table 3.4.

Table 3.4 Categories of the themes support/caring

Nurses' Data	Patients' Data
1. Physical contact and physical closeness	1. A caring relationship
2. Being present through giving time	2. Nurse sparing time to talk
3. Sensitivity and attentiveness to the patient's emotional needs	3. Nurse being understanding about what the patient is going through
4. Physical contact	

The nurses' references to support bear a close similarity to those made by patients about caring. Each group describes the ways in which the nurse who provides care and/or support conveys a proximity to the patient in a variety of ways. These include, for example, 'presence' through close or frequent contact, remaining with and being attentive to the patient and conveying an understanding of the patient's experience. This integration of themes is particularly evident in the patient's accounts.

19. Nurse F (I2: 7) *Support* (This nurse was asked to elaborate on her reference to 'support').

. . . when they are just having things like blood transfusions they really get twitched about it. If you can spend as much time as possible with them; if you can sort of put aside other tasks to sit with them and talk about them or, you know, keep checking . . . they don't need something, they feel less isolated, you know, just somebody to be there.'

20. Nurse A (I1: 24)

'Support is just being in the vicinity of them knowing that you're just there and that you will comfort them if they need it.'

21. Nurse A (I1: 20) *Caring* (elaborating on her reference to 'caring')

'. . . it was an endoscopy he was going in for. I was explaining about that to him and I realised – I thought, he's going to cry in a minute, and I didn't know if it would be better for him if I left the room or if I should stay and comfort him – and tears came before I could decide, so I sort of automatically gave him a big hug, y'know, and said "Oh, I'm sorry you're feeling so miserable" and we sat chatting for quite a bit longer.'

Another ethnographic study of nurses' views of the caring situation identified two of the major themes as 'support as care' and 'presence as care' (Peterson 1985).

The themes of 'caring' and 'support and caring' would seem to occupy a central position in the interim data due to their overlap with all other themes conveying the value of presence. Some of the nurses' accounts on this theme are also incorporated within the dimension the 'presentation of the nurse', but these are not described in this chapter.

22. Patient N (I1: 14)   *A caring relationship*

'. . . if it's a happy what I call a 'caring' relationship, obviously it's good for both the patient and the nurse because they co-operate together.'

23. Patient N (I1: 26–27)   *Nurse being understanding*

'. . . she was caring . . . she understood what I was going through . . . they understand and feel for what you're going through.'

24. Patient L (I1: 16–17)   *Spared time to talk*

'I think just when people err, stop and have time to talk to you – if you've got a problem . . . when they've been busy, you know, and spared time to talk – I think that's a caring thing to do.'

Both empirical and theoretical nursing literature support the notion of support and care as 'presence'. Morrison (1988) reported briefly on an ongoing study of nurses' perceptions of caring, using personal construct theory and involving 25 nurses of charge nurse grade in various clinical settings. One of the constructs identified was 'always has time for the patient'. This is supported by other studies on caring (Brown 1982, Keane 1987).

'Presence' as a construct of caring was identified in Leininger's (1981) ethnoscientific analysis of the perceptions, beliefs and actions of a group of nurses and clients in 30 different cultures, from 1964 to 1981. Details of her data source appear to remain unpublished. Comparison with Leininger's data is limited since it is not specific to any one culture, also, the distinction between nurses' and clients' views are not evident.

A study to explore the lived experience of caring of both nurses and patients by Rieman (1986) and is one of the few to examine beliefs about its consequences for the patient.

The sample of ten non-hospitalised adults had prior inter-actions with a registered nurse. She identified that 'in a caring interaction, the nurse's existential presence is perceived by the client as more than just a physical presence.' This was validated by the informants and is supported by a similar study con-ducted by Forrest (1989). Such physical and mental presence is seen to be available for the client's 'use'. The nurse's caring presence was found to be therapeutic for clients who were helped to feel comfortable, secure, at peace and relaxed.

Some comparisons may also be made between the theoretical literature and the data presented here. Leininger (1977) expressed her belief in caring as a potentially therapeutic act in stating that it is caring that is the most essential ingre-dient to any curative process. This belief is supported by Watson's (1985) theoretical study of caring.

The literature on nurses' views of support is not as exten-sive as that on caring. Also no direct reference has been found to nurses and patient's beliefs in the presence of the nurse as being supportive to the patient. However, Gardener and Wheeler's (1981) inductive study identified 'sitting with patient and spending time' and 'listening' among five most frequently reported aspects of supportive behaviours by nurses, identified in critical incidents; both behaviours could be said to convey a form of 'presence'. In a later study of patients' perceptions of supportive nursing the availability of nurses was the most frequently reported as a requirement for their needs to be met (Gardener and Wheeler 1987).

The availability of the nurse

The nurse's ability or willingness to be available to or give time to attend to the patient's needs is depicted by this theme which is common to both nurses and also patient participants. They describe the difficulty created when it is not possible to give a patient adequate time; particularly in meeting their needs for information and physical assistance. The patients' descrip-tions of the nurse not being available correspond with the nurses' reports of their intent to 'give' or 'spend' time with the patient and the frustration this caused them. This theme represents the recognition by nurses and patient participants groups of the importance of the conditional factors such as time which influence the opportunities the nurse has to benefit the patient.

The patient categories are firstly 'giving time to me' and secondly 'nurses not being available'.

24. Patient L (I1: 16–17)   *Spared time to talk*

'I must've been talking to her for 20 minutes . . . it was different 'cos she was just sat there chatting. She wasn't actually having to do anything, so it was more like a normal conversation . . . rather than someone just there 'cos they're doing something for you.'

25. Patient L (D: 2–3)   *Not enough nurses/being very busy*

'Only five nurses to look after the ward this morning. Usually about 11. Felt really annoyed and frustrated because I wanted a shower and a hairwash but it wasn't possible as they were very busy. The student told me the whole week was going to be like this which didn't make me feel any better. She said she could understand how I felt but I'm sure she couldn't possibly understand the frustration of being dependent and there not being enough people to help.'

The above account shows that difficulty in being available for the patient may reinforce feelings of dependency in the latter.

The two categories in the nurses data, 'having time for the patient' and 'not having time for patients due to the ward being busy' are exemplified in the following accounts.

26. Nurse F (I1: 22)   *Having time for patients*

'I think that quite an important way of affecting someone is letting them have a few minutes of your time. (S: mm) 'cos they all say "you're too busy nurse". I've had people say "can I have a commode – no you're too busy", or, "can I have a word? no you're too busy now I'll ask you later", or "I'll wait", or, "don't bother, don't worry". I think quite a lot of people miss out on care they could've got, by kind of, not taking the opportunity to, kind of, talk with a nurse or doctor, whoever they find useful.'

27. Nurse A (ID: 4)   *Failure to communicate with those patients who have specific communication problems.*

[Overlap with communication theme]

'A while ago we had an Indian lady who spoke no English and had had a stroke and required all care. I think her inability to communicate with us resulted in her receiving pretty inadequate care. Many of our patients, for whatever reason, cannot or find it difficult to communicate and on a busy ward where jobs are having to be skipped, it is likely to be those patients who lose out.'

Some of the nursing literature relevant to this theme has already been described as it relates to other themes depicting the existence and value of the presence of the nurse.

In Altschul's study of nurse-patient interaction in the psychiatric field, open-ended interviews were used to elicit what nursing activities patients found helpful. The nature of the design and setting used by Altschul limit comparison with the data presented here; however, it offers further support for the high value patients place on the nurse's availability.

The precise reasons given for the nurse not being available were often difficult for the participants to identify, however, general statements are made about the nurses being 'very busy' and there being 'not enough nurses'.

A study by Hockey (1976) identified that many nurses were concerned about the shortage of time for their work. Only about a third of the 588 respondents believed that they had enough time. This finding of course gave no indication of the actual quality of care given. When asked what sort of things they would like time for most responded that it would be for communication. Research examining the pattern of verbal interaction between nurse and patient reveals the effect of other influencing factors. Studies in psychiatry (Cormack 1976) and surgical nursing (Macleod-Clarke 1982) both identified that interaction was infrequent, of short duration and typically accompanied nursing activity. It varied with factors such as ward type, time of day, age and social class of patient. Macleod-Clarke warned that patients appear consciously to adopt a passive role, perceiving the nurse as too busy to be worried. The patients may then be reluctant to express their concerns. Whatever the reason for the short duration of nurse-patient interaction the problem of the nurse not being accessible to the patient may be exacerbated by the nurse not communicating her availability to the patient. One of the student nurse participants ('nurse F') reported the value of the nurse communicating her availability to the patient; reference has also been made to this in the literature (Paterson and Zderad 1976).

The nurse: trying to understand the lived experience of illness

'No one had ever understood what the illness meant to this woman before, and the understanding alone was a great gift, because it moved back the walls of isolation and suffering created by the disease.'

(Benner and Wrubel 1989)

Nurse and patient data both convey the importance of the nurse having an awareness of the patient's situation. The corresponding categories are 'sensitivity-insensitivity shown to the patient' (patient) and 'determining what the problem is from the patient's viewpoint and responding to it' (nurses). The nurse's attempts and his or her success in identifying with patient's experience is believed to affect her ability to meet the person's needs.

27. Nurse W (I1: 31–32)   *Determining what the problem is from their (patient's) viewpoint and responding to it.*

'. . . the patients often actually know the problems themselves more than, obviously better than, anybody else. So, if you can determine what the problem is from their point of view, then you can actually treat it in a more effective way.'

28. Nurse A (D: 3)   *Helping a patient to accept that their need is understood and that they are not a nuisance.*

' "B" was extremely worried about the possibility of her needing to keep calling the night staff to fetch her a commode. I sat and listened to her worries and tried to discover *why* it was such a big worry and then tried to make her accept that we understood her need and that to us she was in no way being a nuisance as she felt herself to be.'

In the following accounts the patient describes the restrictions on her autonomy imposed by being wheelchair bound with a chronic neurological disorder, factors which are exacerbated in the hospital environment. Her comments also suggest that an understanding of her situation may be an indirect benefit in that they provide an opportunity for greater rapport with the nurse.

30. Patient L (I1: 62)   *Nurse not being aware of patient's need for space*

'. . . there was just about room for me and there was another table and it was all getting really totally impossible – I just couldn't move in there – really, it was just all too much. I felt quite angry . . . I got upset and tears.'

31. Patient L (I1: 11)   *Recognising the patient's viewpoint*

'. . . nurses who have been in hospital themselves often have a better idea . . . you know what patients are going through, rather than nurses who've never actually experienced help or anything . . . if you've never been in hospital you can't empathise . . . it's just a common ground . . . when you know what it's like to be a patient and to be at the receiving end.'

(I1: 13) . . . it does help to share that sort of experience . . . it's a sort of levelling out . . . a sort of breaking down those sorts of barriers.'

It has been said that while accepting that suffering is personal, and outside the consciousness of other individuals, sufferers may seek a more complete understanding of their suffering from these others (McGilloway and Myco 1985). Although nurses may not be as available as they wish to meet the patient's needs they have opportunities for closeness of contact with patients which allows them to come to know the person. Understanding of illness and treatment from the patient's viewpoint and situation is said to be a central concern of nurses (Wilson-Barnett 1984).

Empathy has been described as a special way of being with another person (Rogers 1975). In most instances it is unclear if the nurse is seen as being sympathetic or empathic. Daniel (1984) distinguishes between the experience of 'like' feelings with sympathy and the development of insight involved in empathy. It is not clear if the nurses' accounts reflect their belief in the value of gaining insight since there is no indication of whether 'like' feelings are experienced by the nurse. This is significant because empathy is considered an essential basis for helping (Carkhuff 1969) and 'as integral to therapeutic nursing' (Gagan 1982). However, the patients' accounts give some indication that it is the nurse's sensitivity to the patient's situation that is seen to be of value.

The value of 'being with' the patient

Aside to the emerging data themes general reference has been made in the literature to the value of the nurse's presence, the act of 'being with' the patient.

Paterson and Zderad (1976) support several themes in saying:

'. . . there is a kind of being, a "being with" or a "being there", this is really a kind of doing for it involves the nurse's active presence. To 'be with' in this fuller sense requires turning one's attention toward the patient, being aware of and open to the here and now shared situation, and communicating one's availability.'

Paterson and Zderad see 'presence' in terms of the nurse being situated in a position from which he or she may relate to the patient and thereby help him or her increase the capacity to make choices. Muetzal's (1988) analysis of the therapeutic relationship between nurse and patient encompasses 'being there' as a feature of the nurse's ability to receive as well as to give. The concept of 'presencing oneself' refers to a person being available to understand and be with another; while physically present with a person one is not preoccupied with other thoughts (Benner and Wrubel 1989). However, it is not entirely clear from the accounts given so far if the nurse's physical presence is accompanied by an attempt to identify with the patient's experience (existential presence).

The image of the nurse as a companion to the patient also conveys 'presence'. Campbell (1984) creates an image of nursing which allows the patient to be given full consideration without distance or manipulation, while protecting the nurse from overwhelming demands. He says '. . . companionship describes a closeness which is neither sexual union nor deep personal friendship. It is a bodily presence which accompanies the other for a while . . . it involves a "being with" and not just a "doing to". ' Companionship helps the person move onward and to encouragement when all seems lost.

Descriptions of the care of people who are dying often describe the value of 'presence'. The fear of death often experienced as the fear of being alone. The wish to avoid isolation and to experience the comfort of having another person present or a spiritual presence, is reflected in the quoted verses from Tennyson's poem. A director of a hospice is quoted as saying that one of the two promises made to their patients is that they will not die alone (Kubler-Ross 1978). Sometimes the need for companionship is set against the desire for the emotional withdrawal from others (Hinton 1972). In a study of the care of a person with progressive tracheal stenosis listening and checking on the patient were seen as qualities of the nurses '. . . being present as people confront life and death and human choices' (Dyck and Benner 1989).

The protective value of 'presence' can be seen from a specific psychological perspective. The concept of 'attachment behaviour' encompasses various forms of behaviour used to attain and/or maintain a desired proximity to another in order to help alleviate anxiety and provide an increased sense of security (Bowlby 1984). Its place in nature to help protect the vulnerable, however, is not confined to infants. Bowlby said that:

> In sickness and calamity, adults often become demanding of others; in conditions of sudden danger or disaster a person will almost certainly seek proximity to another known and trusted person. In such circumstances an increase in attachment behaviour is recognised as natural.

This is supported by Weiss (1982). Bowlby believes that attachment behaviour plays a vital role in adult life, rejecting the claim that it is necessarily regressive.

Although not evident as yet from the data there is a sense in which the presence of the nurse may be found by some to be intrusive. There is sometimes a tension for the suffering person between their need for privacy and the need to be with others. A nurse who has experienced severe depression said:

> To be allowed to escape from company at that particular point in my life was precious indeed, but so was the knowledge that I was not really alone (Altschul 1985).

No conclusions may be drawn as yet from this interim stage of the study, nor is there scope to explore the issues raised so far, however, some of these may be mentioned in conclusion.

It was argued that there is value in exploring the therapeutic effect of nursing through the study of the perspective of nurses and patients, using a qualitative design. This approach has begun to generate concepts and propositions which may illuminate areas of nurse-patient interaction which may be therapeutic in effect. Certainly these elements of a grounded theory developed so far will require a significant degree of refinement before any attempt is made to examine them further using research.

The initial coding of the second stage of fieldwork data indicates that both nurse and patient participants continue to consider the effects of the nurse's presentation and presence on the patient at least, if not more, important than their specific-procedural actions. The presentation of the nurse is the largest dimension of the data for both nurse and patient participants. Therefore, during the continuing analysis categories relating to the importance of the nurse's personal qualities to the patient's welfare will require close examination and comparison with data referring to other aspects of their behaviour. Furthermore, the frequent reference to the influence of the nurse's emotional display also raises questions about the ethics and politics of the use of 'sentimental work' by nurses.

Analysis of the first stage data indicates that there is a fairly high degree of congruence in the behaviour of the nurse believed to affect the patient. However, there are examples of incongruent views such as a nurse's emphasis on the value of giving patients explanations on one ward and a patient's perception that only inappropriate information had been received on the same ward. Such instances serve as important areas for continued analysis.

For discrepancies which appear to be developing between the informants' beliefs about the effect of nurses on patients and the current nursing literature raises at least two important issues: the suitability of the prevailing concept of the 'therapeutic use of self' and the limited reference to nurses as legitimate healers in society.

ACKNOWLEDGEMENTS

The author would like to acknowledge the support and comments of Moira Fordham and the financial assistance of the Nightingale Fund Council, the Tregaski's Bequest (King's College, London) and the Institute of Nursing (Oxford).

REFERENCES

Aamodt, A.M. (1982) 'Examining ethnography for nurse researchers', *West Journal of Nursing Research*, **4**(2), 209–21.

Abercrombie, N., Hill, S. and Turner, B. (1988) *The Penguin Dictionary of Sociology*, Penguin Books, Harmondsworth.

Altschul, A. (1972) *Patient-nurse Interaction: a Study of Interaction Patterns in Acute Psychiatry Wards*, Churchill Livingstone, Edinburgh.

Altschul, A. (1985) 'There won't be a next time', Rippere, V. and Williams, R. (eds.) *Wounded Healers*, John Wiley and Sons Ltd, Chichester.

Argyle, M. and Henderson, M. (1985) *The Anatomy of Relationships*, Heinemann Publishing Ltd, Oxford.

Balint, M. (1964) *The Doctor, His Patient and the Illness*, Pitman, London.

Benner, P. and Wrubel, J. (1989) *The Primacy of Caring: Stress and Coping in Health and Illness*, Addison-Wesley Publishing Company, California.

Blumer, H. (1969) *Symbolic Interactionism: Perspective and Method*, Prentice-Hall, New Jersey.

Bowlby, J. (1984) *Attachment and Loss: volume 1, Attachment*, Penguin Books, Harmondsworth.

Brown, L. (1982) 'Behaviours of Nurses perceived by Hospitalised Patients as Indicators of Care', (Doctoral dissertation, University of Colorado, Boulder) *Dissertation Abstracts International*, **43**, 4361B (University microfilms # DA8209803)

Burgess, R.G. (1984) *In the Field: an Introduction to Field Research*, Allen & Unwin, London.

Campbell, A.V. (1984) *Moderated Love: a Theory or Professional Care*, SPCK, London.

Carkhuff, R.R. (1969) *Helping and Human Relations: a Primer for Lay Helpers.* Volumes 1 and 2, Holt Rinehart and Winston, New York.

Chapman, G. (1983) 'Ritual and rational action in hospitals', *Journal of Advanced Nursing*, **81** 13–20.

Chapman, G. (1986) Social action theory and psychosocial nursing' in Kennedy, R., Heymans, A., and Tischler, L. (eds.) *The Family as In-Patient: Families and Adolescents at the Cassel Hospital*, Free Association Books, London.

Chenitz, W.C. and Swanson, J.M. (1986) *From Practice to Grounded Theory: Qualitative Research in Nursing*, Addison-Wesley Publishing, California.

Corbin, J. (1986) 'Coding writing memos, and diagramming' in Chenitz, W.C. and Swanson, J.M. (eds.) (see above).

Cormack, D. (1976) *Psychiatric Nursing Observed*, Royal College of Nursing, London.

Cuff, E.C. and Payne, G.C.F. (eds.) (1984) *Perspectives in Sociology*, Allen & Unwin, London.

Daniel, J. (1984) 'Sympathy' or 'empathy' (letter to the editor) *Journal of Medical Ethics*, **10**(2), 103.

Duck, S. (1984) *Personal Relationships 5: Repairing Personal Relationships*, Academic Press, London.

Dyck, B. and Senner, P. (1989) 'Dialogues with excellence: the paper crane', *American Journal of Nursing*, **89**(8), 824–5.

Ersser, S. (1988) 'Nursing beds and nursing therapy' in Pearson, A. (ed.) *Primary Nursing: Nursing in the Burford and Oxford Nursing Development Units* Croom Helm, London.

Field, P.A. and Morse, J.M. (1985) *Nursing Research: The Application of Qualitative Approaches*, Croom Helm, London.

Forrest, D. (1989) 'The experience of caring', *Journal of Advanced Nursing*, **14** 815–23.

Gagan, J.M. (1982) 'Methodological notes on empathy' *Advanced Nursing Science*, **5**(2) 65–72.

Gardner, K.G. and Wheeler, E.C. (1981) 'Nurses' perceptions of the meaning of support issues', *Mental Health Nursing*, **3** 13–28.

Gardner, K.G. and Wheeler, E.C. (1987) Patients' perceptions of support *Western Journal of Nursing Research*, **9**(1) 115–31.

Germain, C. (1986) 'Ethnography: the method' in Munhall, P.L. and Oller, C.J. *Nursing Research: A Qualitative Perspective*, Appleton-Century-Crofts, Norwalk.

Glaser, B. (1978) *Theoretical Sensitivity*, Sociology Press, California.

Glaser, B. and Strauss, A. (1967) *The Discovery of Grounded Theory*, Aldine, Chicago.

Goffman, E. (1971) *The Presentation of Self in Everyday Life*, Pelican Books, Harmondsworth.

Gow, K.M. (1982) *How Nurses' Emotions Affect Patient Care: Self Studies by Nurses*, Springer Publishing Company, New York.

Hamkin, C. (1987) *Research Design: Strategies and Choices in the Design of Social Research*, Allen & Unwin, London.

Hall, L. (1969) The Loeb Center for Nursing and Rehabilitation, Montefiore Hospital and Medical Center, Bronx, New York. *International*

Journal of Nursing Studies, **6**, 81–95.
Hammersley, M. and Atkinson, P. (1983) *Ethnography: Principles and Practice*, Tavistock Publications, London.
Harré, R. and Secord, P.F. (1972) *The Explanation of Social Behaviour*, Basil Blackwell, Oxford.
Hinton, J. (1982) *Dying*, Penguin Books Ltd, Harmondsworth.
Hochschild, A.R. (1983) *The Managed Heart: Commercialisation of Human Feeling*, University of California Press, Berkeley.
Hockey, L. (1976) *Woman in Nursing*, Hodder & Stoughton, London.
Hockey, L. 1989) 'Therapeutic nursing: its development and debut'. Unpublished paper, National Conference on Therapeutic Nursing, St Catherine's College, Oxford.
Jourard, S. (1971) *The Transparent Self*, Van Nostrand Reinhold Co. Inc., New York.
Keane, S.M. (1987) Caring: nurse-patient perceptions, *Rehabilitation Nursing*, **12**(4) 182–4 and 187.
Kubler-Ross, E. (1978) *To Live Until We Say Goodbye*, Prentice Hall Inc. Englewood Cliffs, New Jersey.
Leininger, M.M. (1977) 'Caring: the essence and central focus of nursing', *American Nurses Foundation (Nursing Research Report)* **12**(1).
Leininger, M.M. (1981) *Caring: an essential Human Need. Proceedings of Three National Caring Conferences*, C.B. Stack, Inc. New Jersey.
Leininger, M.M. (1985) *Qualitative Research Methods in Nursing*, Grune & Stratton, Inc., Orlando.
Lofland, J. (1971) *Analysing Social Situations: A Guide to Qualitative Observation and Analysis*, Wadsworth Publishing Co. Inc., Belmont, California.
Macleod-Clarke, J. (1982) 'Nurse-Patient Interaction. An Analysis of Conversations on Surgical Wards', Unpublished Ph.D Thesis, University of London.
McGilloway, O. and Myco, F. (1985) *Nursing and Spiritual Care*, Harper & Row, London.
Meleis, A.I. (1985) *Theoretical Nursing: Development and Progress*, J.B. Lippincott Co., Philadelphia.
Mellow, J. (1966) 'Nursing therapy as a treatment and clinical investigative approach to mental illness', *Nursing Forum*, **3**(5) 64–73.
Morrison, P. (1988) 'Nurses perceptions of caring' *Nursing Times (Short Report)*, **84**(9) p. 51.
Muetzal, P.A. (1988) 'Therapeutic nursing' in Pearson, A. (ed.) *Primary Nursing: Nursing in the Burford and Oxford Nursing Development Unit*, Croom Helm, London.
Orem, D. (1980) *Nursing: Concepts of Practice*, McGraw-Hill, New York.
Paterson, J.G. and Zderad, L.T. (1976) *Humanistic Nursing*, John Wiley & Sons, New York.
Pearson, A., Durand, I. and Punton, S. (1988) *Therapeutic Nursing: an Evaluation of an Experimental Nursing Unit in the British National Health Service*, Nursing Development Units, Burford and Oxford.
Peplau, H. (1952) *Interpersonal Relations in Nursing* Putnam, New York.
Peterson, B.H. (1985) 'A qualitative account and analysis of a care situation', in Leininger, M. op. cit.

Ragguci, A.T. (1972) 'The ethnographic approach to nursing research', *Nursing Research*, **21**(6) 485–90.

Rieman, D.J. (1986) 'The essential structure of a caring interaction: doing phenomenology' in Munhall, P. and Oiler, C. *Nursing Research: A Qualitative Perspective*, Appleton-Century-Crofts, Norwalk.

Rogers, C.R. (1975) 'Empathic: an unappreciated way of being', *Counselling Psychologist*, **21** 95–103.

Schwartz, L.H. and Schwartz, J.L. (1972) *The Psychodynamics of Patient Care*, Prentice Hall, Inc., New Jersey.

Smith, P. (1988) 'The emotional labour of nursing', *Nursing Times*, **84**(44) 50–1.

Spradley, J. (1979) *The Ethnographic Interview*, Holt, Rinehart & Winston, Chicago.

Stimpson, G. (1975) *Going to See the Doctor: The Consultation Process in General Practice*, Routledge & Kegan Paul, London.

Stockwell, F. (1972) *The Unpopular Patient*, Royal College of Nursing, London.

Strauss, A., Fagerhaugh, S., Suezek, B., and Wiener, C. (1982) 'Sentimental work in technological hospitals', *Sociology of Health and Illness*, **4**(3) 254–78.

Taylor, C.M. (1982) *Mereness' Essentials of Psychiatric Nursing* (11th edn), C.V. Mosby Co., St. Louis.

Tennyson, A. (1986) 'Be near me when the sensuous frame' in Benn, J. *Memorials*, Ravette, Horsham.

Travelbee, J. (1971) *Interpersonal Aspects of Nursing* (2nd ed.) F.A. Davis, Philadelphia.

Uys, L.R. (1980) 'Towards the development of an operational definition of the concept 'therapeutic use of self', *International Journal of Nursing Studies* **17**(3) 175–80.

Weber, M. (1978) in Roth, G., Wittich, C. *Economy and Society: an Outline of Interpretive Sociology* (2 vols) (Translated by Fischoff)), University of California Press, California.

Watson, J. (1985) *The Philosophy and Science of Caring*, Colorado Association University Press, Colorado.

Weddel, D. (1968) 'Change of approach' in Barnes, P. (ed.) *Psychosocial Nursing: Studies from the Cassel Hospital*, Tavistock Publications Ltd., London.

Weiss, R.S. (1982) 'Attachment in adult life', in Parkes, C.M. and Stevenson-Hinde, J. (eds) *The Place of Attachment in Human Behaviour*, Basic Books, New York.

Wilson-Barnett, J. (1984) 'Key functions in nursing', The 1984 Winifred Raphael Memorial Lecture. Royal College of Nursing, London.

Wilson-Barnett, J. and Carrigy, A. (1978) Factors affecting patients responses to hospitalisation. *Journal of Advanced Nursing*, **3**(3) 221–8.

Chapter 4

Patient education in therapeutic nursing

BARBARA VAUGHAN

No man can reveal to you aught but that which lies half asleep in the dawning of your knowledge.
Gibran (1926) *The Prophet* on speaking of teaching.

The importance of patient education in therapeutic nursing is now widely acknowledged and is implicit, if not explicit, in the majority of conceptual or theoretical frameworks of nursing which are found in the literature. For example there is no way in which nurses can help patients to maximise their ability to self care as advocated by Orem (1980) unless they share information with them. Indeed Orem describes teaching as one of the essential nursing acts. Similarly there is a fundamental need to become involved in patient education in Roy's (1984) notion of helping patients to adapt to stresses, King's (1981) theory of goal attainment or Roper et al.'s (1985) ideas about independence. Neuman (1982) goes so far as to advocate that care planning be divided into primary, secondary and tertiary components, the first being concerned with preventative factors, the second with dealing with an acute phase of ill health and the third with helping patients to prevent recurrence. The implications for teaching are self evident in such an approach but particularly conspicuous in the primary and tertiary phases of care.

The rise in awareness about health education has also become a topic which has attracted many nurses working both clinically and in research as they recognise this need which has been so widely neglected to date. While this fundamental contribution to health care may not be the sole province of nurses there is certainly a major contribution which they can make. Yet again there is a suggestion that the teaching function of the nurse must be acknowledged and developed if he or she is to be able to work effectively as a health educator.

According to Watson (1985) nurses have always maintained that teaching about health is one of the main functions of nursing. She suggests that this is one of the criteria which may differentiate 'professional nursing' from 'technical nursing', commenting that:

> 'The amount and level of teaching done by a nurse who has a baccalaureate or masters degree is expected to be greater than the amount done by a nurse who has a diploma or associate degree. Patients/clients as well as health professionals expect that.'

It is interesting to speculate how easily such a comment transfers from the expectations of an American society to another culture such as the UK. Nurses with degrees or higher degrees are still in the minority in many countries. Furthermore there is, as yet, little evidence to suggest that the general public acknowledge nurses as credible sources of information. Furthermore the sharing of knowledge which is implicit in such a statement does not comply with the traditional view of professions who, it can be suggested, maintain part of their status by retaining a 'mystical body of knowledge' (Friedson 1975). Such a stance would be antithetical to therapeutic nursing where partnership with patients and sharing of knowledge is crucial. Alternatively, however, there is an implication in Watson's words that there is a depth of knowledge in nursing which is commensurate with studying to higher degree levels and, more importantly, studying to this level should enhance the practising skills of the nurse. Such thoughts go some way to offering a sound rationale for the current move in nurse education to diploma level since if patient teaching is a core part of practice it cannot be achieved effectively without advanced knowledge of health and nursing, which would include knowledge of learning and teaching theories. Furthermore her words could be taken as a guide or indicator to some of the criteria which could be used in evaluating nursing in terms of both the skills required and the service which nurses offer.

TEACHING AND LEARNING – THE STATE OF THE ART

If it is accepted that teaching is a part of nursing then the fundamental questions which have to be addressed relate to how both nurses and patients perceive teaching and learning. It is not the intention within this chapter to give detailed explanations of theories of teaching and learning since they are widely available elsewhere (e.g. Knowles et al. 1984, Bigge 1976, Rogers 1983). It is, however, important to ensure that there is a common understanding of what is meant by these terms.

Teaching

Wilson-Barnett (1989) describes patient teaching as 'the process of increasing patients' or clients' understanding about their state of health, disease, treatment and rehabilitation by giving information in a planned and structured way'. However in nursing much of the teaching which occurs is aimed at helping people to manage their own lives more independently. Thus it can be argued that helping patients/clients to increase their theoretical understanding of what is happening to them is only the beginning of the process. What is even more vital is that the teaching occurs in such a way that it is meaningful to the recipients in making decisions about any changes in their way of life which may be beneficial to their health and which they *wish to make*. It is, of course, much more difficult to interpret knowledge in this way so that it can be of practical use to the learner and requires much more skilful teaching.

Such difficulties are widely understood by nurses themselves as evidence grows of the well known theory/practice gap. As far back as the mid 1970s Bendall (1975) gave stark evidence of the lack of correlation between what nurses said they did and what they actually did. In the same way while patients may learn new facts about different things which could affect their health status this does not mean to say that those facts can be easily transferred into a change of behaviour. Thus teaching undertaken by nurses must go well beyond the simple imparting of new knowledge to an assurance that the patients/clients have not only absorbed that knowledge but also found a way of making use of it in managing their own lives.

Facilitating learning

Some people have rejected the use of the term 'teaching', since to many it has implications of an expert passing on knowledge to a pupil. Rogers (1983) for example suggests that he has no use for a word which implies imparting knowledge or skill to another, and prefers to use the term 'facilitating learning' and this phrase has been widely adopted by others. Indeed its use may be justified if teaching is confined solely to helping people to learn new facts about a given topic whether the topic is their own health or anything else. However, if teaching is taken more broadly as providing the facilities under which another may learn then maybe Rogers' view is a little harsh since there are times when it is entirely appropriate for an expert to share his or her knowledge with another. The difference may be in what the expert expects the recipient actually to do with the knowledge. If the expectation is that the recipient will accept the information in blind faith then maybe such an approach can be criticised. If however there is an understanding of sharing and debate about the relevance of that knowledge to a given person at a given point in his or her life then it can be argued that teaching is entirely appropriate.

What can be called to question is the style of teaching which is used to impart knowledge from one person to another. While it has already been argued that 'didactic' teacher-led lectures can, in fact, have a contribution to make in patient/client education there is also a case to be made for nurses having sufficient discrimination to know both the advantages and the limitations of such an approach. What has to be remembered is that not every person has the same learning styles and while some people find a degree of safety and group support in the more impersonal and anonymous formal learning situation, others will find that same impersonal approach unhelpful. Thus, as in all other areas of nursing, practitioners need to have sufficient knowledge not only of their specific subject area but also of the variations in peoples' learning styles in order to be able to practice well.

Experiential learning

Following a humanistic approach Carl Rogers (1969) suggests

strongly that for learning to be effective the drive and impetus must come from the learner him/herself. In defining significant or experiential learning he has identified the essential elements as:

1. *A quality of personal involvement* – the whole person in both his feeling and cognitive aspects being *in* the learning event.
2. *It is self initiated* – Even when the impetus comes from the outside the sense of discovery, of reaching out, of grasping and comprehending comes from within.
3. *It is pervasive* – it makes a difference in the behaviour, the attitudes, perhaps even the personality of the learner.
4. *It is evaluated by the learner* – He knows whether it is meeting his needs, whether it leads towards what he wants to know, whether it illuminates the dark area of ignorance he is experiencing.

Inherent in Rogers' view of learning is the humanistic belief that there is potential in all people to develop and grow and that by facilitating learning a teacher can help in this process. However unless there is personal commitment and involvement within the learner, efforts to help are fruitless.

Experiential learning has gained considerable interest in recent years particularly in helping people to develop the human skills of self knowledge or self awareness. Burnard (1985) sees it as a valuable way of helping nurses to learn these skills which according to Peplau (1952) and many others since, are a prerequisite to therapeutic nursing. The argument is that without knowledge of self one cannot empathise with others in order to help them to learn from new experiences.

Burnard (1985) suggests that learning can occur both through current experiences and from past experiences, the emphasis always being on action. Some of his suggestions which are primarily aimed at nurse education may be equally applicable for patient education. For example *recall* (an intentional action) of a previous hospital admission may help a patient to understand his or her fears of a current hospital admission. Similarly giving patients the opportunity to handle their own drugs and self medicate prior to discharge from hospital (a positive action) may lead to a better understanding of the need to continue taking the drugs and more accuracy in their use following discharge.

While the use of experiential learning methods can be of great value to nurses it is also necessary to add a word of warning. Many people, but particularly those who underwent their general education a long time ago, will not be familiar with experiential methods of learning, their recall of a teacher being someone who told them what was 'right and proper'. Indeed they may have an expectation that it is the responsibility of health care workers to 'tell me what is good for me' without apparently being concerned with the reasons why. Furthermore, some people find the very involvement of some experiential learning methods extremely uncomfortable and disconcerting. This does not mean to say that they cannot be employed when working with patients. It does however raise a note of caution again in the importance of matching teaching methods to the individual needs of patients rather than becoming over-enthusiastic about a particular approach which may not be right for everyone.

An unconditional service

A further note of warning concerns the way in which nurses themselves feel about this approach to learning. Because of their expert knowledge and their privileged position of access to personal information about patients, there may be times when they feel that a patient's own actions are harmful and *should* be stopped. Thus they can feel an obligation to try to influence a patient's behaviour when the patient is neither motivated nor ready to learn. If Rogers' thesis is accepted, such actions are unlikely to have a lasting effect. Furthermore it has to be added that in some instances patients are censored for non-compliance regardless of the underlying circumstances. This raises an interesting issue that nurses have a responsibility to offer an unconditional service. There are some who believe that if a patient's own actions are not appropriate then the obligation of the health care worker to offer a service is no longer applicable, the obvious example being of someone who continues to smoke despite being given information about its harmful effects. The question which has to be raised is whether the service which nurses offer is, in fact, unconditional. There is a need for nurses themselves to have self knowledge of how they feel about such situations. Working with a patient in anger and resentment is unlikely to be effective yet there are times when these feelings are very real. There is no easy answer to dilemmas of this kind which nurses face so often. However it does raise very important issues of their own learning needs, maybe using experiential methods of reflection and debate in order that they may increase their understanding of themselves and therefore hopefully their skills in supporting patients through using appropriate learning methods which are geared to individual needs.

ALTERNATIVE APPROACHES

Watson (1985) suggests that the 'tutorial' method of teaching is probably the one which is seen most commonly in clinical practice where teaching is an isolated event in the pattern of care on offer. However she also advocates the promotion of what she calls 'interpersonal teaching/learning' as a major caring factor. In this instance the interaction can be seen as a much more personal experience with growth and under-standing occurring for both the nurse and the patient. Teaching and learning in this sense go well beyond the traditional expectations of an expert imparting knowledge to a learner about a specific isolated event. In this situation both parties will play the roles of both teacher and learner throughout their interaction. Thus the nurse will learn from the patient of past experiences, previous coping strategies or personal perceptions of a given situation while in his or her turn the nurse will share both cognitive and perceptual information which may help the patient/client to manage his or her own health. In turn both parties have the opportunity to develop their understanding of a situation and extend the repertoire of information which they can use to problem solve both currently and in the future.

This view of nursing, as a developmental process in which both patient and nurse grow, was described by Peplau (1952) as far back as the early 1950s. However she argues that there is a difference in the way in which peers may learn together and the way in which a nurse and a client will both develop. She describes the relationship between a skilled nurse and a client as one of 'professional closeness' where the nurse has developed sufficient empathy to be able to manage her own behaviour in such a way as to help a client to develop and learn through a personal health crisis. Such a relationship is differentiated from interpersonal closeness where the needs of each party take mutual precedence, physical closeness of a more personal nature and pseudo-closeness where false sympathy can deny true empathy and be used as a barrier to professional support by the nurse (Peplau 1969). With professional closeness one of the major functions of nursing can be seen as the creation of environments in which clients can feel safe and learn more about themselves which can be of both short- and long-term benefit to them. This does not, however, negate the fact that in each new nursing situation the nurse will also learn something new which can be added to her total repertoire of knowledge for future practice.

Ideas such as this comply well with the way in which Benner (1984) has identified levels of nursing competence ranging from that of a novice to an expert practitioner. Using a care study example she describes how the expert practitioner, who has gained advanced formal knowledge as well as a wealth of practical experience, is not only able to recognise the learning needs of a patient but also the *time* at which that patient is most ready to learn. It is her premiss that the less experienced nurse, while knowing what it is that she should be teaching, will be much less skilled in knowing when and how to share information.

The reasoning behind this view is partly based on the fact that until any nurse has a considerable length of experience in a given situation she is not able to be sufficiently sensitive to the cues to be able to react to individual differences between people. She therefore has to rely more heavily on either formal theories or personal life experiences which cannot be the same as those of the person with whom he or she is working. Thus if she knows that information can lead to a reduction in stress her major goal will be to share that information regardless of the contextual circumstances, particularly if she has found this approach helpful on a personal level. There are, however, some instances when sharing of information at the wrong time can make a situation more, rather than less, stressful. It is the mark of an expert to be able to discern not only what to tell but when to tell it.

The skill of making judgements of this kind takes patient education well beyond the realms of routine practice and reinforces Watson's premiss of relating the degree and depth of teaching with which a nurse is involved with her level of education, provided that the formal education is matched with advanced clinical experience.

Teaching and stress reduction

There is now a considerable body of knowledge supporting the notion that patient education can lead to a reduction in stress levels in patients, thus enhancing their recovery. Limited information, on the other hand, can lead to a feeling of lack of control which in its turn can lead to a feeling of helplessness stress. While this principle has been well accepted in some areas of care, such as before surgery (Boore 1978, Hayward 1975), it is questionable as to how widely it is accepted in other areas. For example, it is not unusual for patients to know that they will be having some form of investigation on a given day but not to know the time. In consequence there is no way that they can plan their own day with regard to simple things such as visiting the shop or even going to the bathroom, for fear of being absent at the crucial moment when they are needed. Waiting seems to be the order of the day. Such conditions are not accepted by most people in other circumstances in their lives and can give rise to considerable annoyance yet they are commonplace in health care.

While it is often not possible to know the exact time of forthcoming events it is sometimes feasible to give people some explanation of the need for delay or waiting which may reduce the amount of anxiety or anger they feel. For example, there is anecdotal evidence that there seems to be less disturbance in the waiting area of an accident department if people know the reason for the delay such as the fact that an emergency is being dealt with elsewhere. Similarly there are times when all people need to know is that they will not 'miss their turn' if they disappear to the bathroom for a few minutes, provided that they let someone know where they will be. It is often just a case of saying that it is all right to do these things, of 'giving permission' and freeing people to do things for themselves rather than having to wait passively and compliantly for things to happen to them. Actions of this kind may seem to be simplistic and obvious but in reality they are often omitted, simply because the need for information has not been recognised. Furthermore they do not fall into the formal category of health care teaching since they are not directly related to a specific health problem. However it is often small things such as these which become the focus of attention and cause the greatest worries. Waiting and boredom are common factors which people complain about when they are receiving health care, which can all add to the total accumulation of stress.

In talking of interpersonal teaching/learning Watson (1985) has identified factors, supported by research from the psychosocial fields as well as from clinical studies which suggest that information:

'. . . promotes accurate expectations and reduces discomforting discrepancies between the degree of stress expected and the degree of stress experienced.

. . . increases the ability to predict what will happen, leading to a feeling of being in control, and reducing associated fears.

. . . fosters the realistic worry and mental rehearsal necessary for emotional acceptance of stress.

. . . changes beliefs and reduces the dreadful fantasies that may be caused by the impending stress.

. . . leads to information that may constitute a method of dealing with the illness and conceptualising it in a less stressful way.

. . . is intimately involved in the evaluation of situations as threatening and the evaluation of ways of reducing threat.'

In reviewing these factors it is interesting to see how familiar they are to most people in their everyday lives and are not unique to health care situations. Feeling out of control because one does not know what is happening is a common enough experience to most of us and it often arises out of simple lack of information. Furthermore how many people have discovered that the fantasy of a dreaded trip to the dentist, often arising from unreal worries, was not nearly as bad in reality. Our imaginations can play disconcerting tricks at times.

There is some evidence to suggest that sharing information prior to an event can, in fact, increase the initial amount of anxiety experienced (e.g. Wilson-Barnet 1978) and some people have used this as a reason for not talking with patients about what will happen. However to counter this argument there is also considerable evidence to suggest that if people do not undergo the 'work of worry' prior to an event their actual experience of that event is considerably worse at the time as they are unprepared for what will happen (Janis 1974). If they are unrealistic about the forthcoming event, for example not acknowledging that surgery will cause a degree of pain, then the actual pain experience can come as a much greater shock and be more difficult to manage. Without prior knowledge people are not in a position to prepare coping strategies from their repertoire of past experience. While a caregiver may be able to make suggestions of ways in which stressful situations could be coped with it is only the individual himself who will know what has worked for him personally in past situations. For example it is customary to use opiates in the management of postoperative pain but there is now a growing number of people who prefer to reduce the amount of analgesia taken and use relaxation or distraction to help themselves. If there is no knowledge that pain may occur then such actions cannot be prepared for.

In the same way there may be others who have extreme fantasies about the degree of pain they will have to undergo following surgery. In this situation false promises that there will be no pain can be just as harmful as leaving the patients with their fantasies. But honest discussion about the degree of pain and the strategies which can be employed to control it can only be helpful. Furthermore patients/clients may justifiably lose faith in those who are trying to help them if they are perceived as less than honest.

Teaching and quality of life

The degree of disruption which people will accept in their daily lives because of a health care difficulty is a constant source of amazement. Yet in many instances patient education can make a significant difference to the way in which they can adapt to either short- or long-term disabilities. For example in early data collection in a study relating to information given to patients prior to discharge following surgery one highly intelligent patient reported that he had not had a bath for two weeks (it was the height of summer) because no one had told him that it didn't matter too much if he got his wound wet.

While in the long term this would not affect his recovery from surgery, in the short term it would make a considerable difference to the quality of his everyday life! In the follow-up to this study there was very positive response from patients who had been given written information supported by personal teaching of how to cope at home in the early days following surgery (Vaughan 1988).

Similarly Pearson (1987) has found that if people are given written information with suggestions about how they can adapt their lifestyles when wearing a below knee plaster their degree of independence in activities of daily living is significantly enhanced. Even more importantly, in his study of nursing beds Pearson found that independence in living was considerably higher at the time of discharge and at a point six weeks after discharge in those patients who had been cared for in a unit where therapeutic teaching was fundamental to nursing practice (Pearson et al. 1989). This important study goes some way to demonstrating the vital contribution which nurses can make to the welfare of patients, measurable more in terms of the quality of their lifestyles indicated by their ability to be independent and to have some say in the control of their own lives, than in actual care.

Teaching and personal growth

Much has already been said about the way in which sharing of information, teaching, or facilitation of learning can enhance the lives of both patients and nurses. However it is also important to recognise that this is not an easy thing to achieve. Inherent in the notion of teaching and learning is the need to change since 'unused' new knowledge is fruitless. However change requires energy and commitment. It is, in many instances, easier to maintain the 'status quo' than to introduce a new order of things. Suggestions of change can pose personal threats to individuals as well as creating a fear of the unknown, of failure or of error of judgement.

The action of sharing or imparting information to others and of giving people choice in how they handle that information on a personal basis can, in itself, be a threat to the power of the holder. Basically it means that there is a shift in control of what happens from the person who holds the resources, in this instance knowledge gained through professional education, to the recipient. Similarly there is a shift away from a model of creating dependency to one of creating a greater degree of independence. While there is considerable emphasis laid on the importance of nurses in helping patients to gain independence, there are still some who see nursing as caring and interpret caring as doing things *for* others. In reality this is far from the truth.

Thus sharing knowledge with patients not only puts nurses in a position of having less control than has been the case in the past but, in many instances, asks them to make fundamental differences in the way in which they practise. It has already been said that lack of control is one of the factors which create stress in patients and it has to be acknowledged that the same holds true for nurses themselves. However stress does not always have to be seen in negative terms. Instead it can be seen as the necessary stimulus to growth, provided that support is given during the period of development and learning, which for a professional practitioner should continue throughout his or her career. Access to both continuing education and support groups on either a formal or an informal basis become vital to good practice since it can be suggested that nurses cannot be asked to care for patients unless they are cared for too.

Pre-requisites to therapeutic teaching

It is sad to reflect that while there is a huge amount of evidence to support the fact that sharing knowledge with patients can make a considerable difference not only to the degree of stress which they experience but also to their ability to live independently, teaching is still not an everyday activity in clinical practice. This raises questions as to why such a situation should have arisen. Unfortunately it can be suggested that a large number of nurses do not acknowledge the extent and importance of their teaching function. When priorities have to be set in a busy clinical setting it is often the case that 'visible work' gets done at the cost of the less visible but arguably more important invisible work of helping people to learn. There also appears to be some confusion of who is responsible for what. A small study carried out with nurses working with leukaemic patients highlighted that, while nurses acknowledged that they were in the best position to teach patients about both their clinical condition and ways of adjusting their lifestyles, they neither felt it was their responsibility nor had the knowledge to do so. They did not perceive health education, the focus of this study, as part of their role (Preston 1988).

A further concern is that, to date, knowledge about teaching and learning have not played a high profile in the curriculum for basic nurse education, these skills often being 'tagged on' either as part of a post basic course or as a separate learning activity. In this instance the emphasis is often on teaching students rather than patients. Hopefully this situation will improve with the development of our own understanding of the relevance of patient teaching in nursing and the development of a new curriculum but this still leaves the vast body of nurses already in practice and emphasises the essential need for continuing education.

So what are the areas in which a nurse requires competence in order to participate effectively in patient teaching? Ellis (1989) has suggested that many practitioners work from an 'understanding within the privacy of one's own head' and suggests that they 'survive in practice through the application of imperfectly articulated intuitive knowledge'. While the importance of intuition should never be denied such a position is unacceptable if knowledge is to be shared with others. Thus the first pre-requisite to teaching is an in-depth understanding of the subject to be taught. As Manthey (1980) suggests, for nurses this is not confined to matters which can be clearly classified as nursing, but also requires a clear understanding of the disease processes which are affecting the patient. This does not mean that nurses need to have the depth of knowledge which doctors have in relationship to disease. What it does mean is that they require a working knowledge of the disease processes which may affect the specific client group with whom they work since lack of understanding about the aetiology and prognosis of the disease and the possible courses of treatment would lead to a danger of false or unhelpful teaching. For example teaching skills of mobility to someone who has a progressive motor neurone disease will be quite different from working with someone who is paraplegic but whose clinical condition is not likely to alter or deteriorate.

A second area of competence for the expert practitioner lies in developing an understanding of the way in which people learn. Such knowledge will guide them, not only in deciding what to teach but also in using their clinical discretion in making decisions about when and where to teach it. Linked with this is a knowledge of how to teach. Having expert knowledge alone is not the same as being able to share that knowledge with others. Indeed we have all suffered from time to time as a result of experts using terms with which we are not familiar, making false assumptions of what we already know, or moving on to a new topic too quickly for us to be able to grasp a new concept. There are skills in teaching which, like most other things, can be learned, and to rely on skills with which one is born is not sufficient. Thus both learning and teaching become key components in any basic nursing curriculum.

Finally if it is accepted that teaching is an interpersonal activity occurring between two or more people rather than simply an expert passing on knowledge didactically, then it becomes essential that teachers develop self knowledge. Without exploring how as an individual the world around us is perceived and interacted with on a personal basis it is unlikely that help can be offered to others.

CONCLUSION

The arguments which have been put forward in this chapter are that patient education in therapeutic nursing goes well beyond the realms of didactic teaching and is, in fact, an integral part of everyday nursing. While it has been suggested that there is a legitimate place for 'experts to teach' the process is in fact much more complex than simply imparting knowledge to another since if that knowledge is not seen as being relevant or important it will not be understood. Furthermore in any teaching situation learning can and should occur for all the people concerned including the so-called teacher. Thus it is not seen as a separate and isolated function but an integral part of practice.

For the future it has been suggested that there are two paths which nurses could follow (Orlando 1987). They may choose to extend their roles along a path of advanced technology and enhance their skills in attaining ever more complex technical skills. In this instance maybe teaching has a lesser part to play as the role would become essentially technical in nature and dependent on medicine. Alternatively there is an option to expand the nursing function of working with people to assist them in the management of their own lives by helping them to gain a greater understanding of the knowledge and skills which will equip them to live independently. Here there is a clear independent function of nursing. If this is the case then patient education is an essential component of therapeutic nursing. Much work is still needed in developing our understanding of how patient education in therapeutic nursing can help others to develop and grow but if the belief in the value of this work is upheld it is a path well worth exploring.

REFERENCES

Bendall, E. (1975) *So You Passed Nurse* Royal College of Nursing, London.

Benner, P. (1984) *From Novice to Expert – Excellence and Power in Clinical Nursing Practice*, Addison Wesley Publishing Co., California.

Bigge, M. (1975) *Learning Theories for Teachers* (3rd edn), Harper and Row Publishers, London.

Boore, J. (1978) *Prescription for Recovery*, Royal College of Nursing, London.

Burnard, P. (1985) *Learning Human Skills – a Guide for Nurses*, Heinemann Publishing Group Ltd., Oxford.

Ellis, R. (1989) *Professional Competence and Quality Assurance in the Caring Professions*, Chapman and Hall, London.

Friedson, E. (1975) *Profession of Medicine*, Dodd, Mead and Co., New York.

Hayward, J. (1975) *Information – A Prescription Against Pain*, Royal College of Nursing, London.

Janis, I.L. (1974) *Psychological Stress*, Academic Press, New York.

King, I.M. (1981) *Toward a Theory of Nursing*, John Wiley & Sons Ltd., New York.

Knowles, (1973) *The Adult Learner – a Neglected Species*, Gulf Publishing Co., London.

Knowles *et al.* (1984) *Androgogy in Action – Applying Modern Principles of Adult Learning*, Jossey Bass, San Francisco.

Manthey, M. (1980) *Primary Nursing*, Blackwell Scientific Press, Oxford.

Neuman, B. (1982) *The Neuman Systems Model*, Appleton-Century-Crofts, Norwalk, Connecticut.

Orem, D. (1980) *Nursing – Concepts of Practice* (2nd edn), McGraw-Hill, New York.

Orlando, I. (1987) 'Nursing in the 21st century – alternative paths' *Journal of Advanced Nursing*, **12**(4) 405–12.

Pearson, A. (1987) *Living in a Plaster*, Royal College of Nursing, London.

Pearson, A., Durand, I. and Punton, S. (1989) 'Determining quality in a unit where nursing is the primary intervention', *Journal of Advanced Nursing*, 269–73.

Peplau, H. (1952) *Interpersonal Relations in Nursing*, G.P. Putman, New York.

Peplau, H. (1969) 'Professional closeness' *Nursing Forum*, **8**(4), 342–60.

Preston, R. (1988) *Nurses as Health Educators*, Burford Nursing Development Unit.

Rogers, C. (1969) *Freedom to Learn*, Bell and Howell, Ohio.

Rogers, C. (1983) *Freedom to Learn for the Eighties*, Merrill, Ohio.

Roper, N., Logan, W. and Tiernay, A. (1985) *The Elements of Nursing* (2nd edn), Churchill Livingstone, Edinburgh.

Roy, C. (1976) *Introduction to Nursing – an Adaptation Model*, Prentice Hall, Old Tappin, New Jersey.

Vaughan, B. (1988) 'Homeward bound discharge following surgery' *Nursing Times*, April 13th, **84**(15), 28–33.

Watson, J. (1985) *The Philosophy and Science of Nursing*, Associated University Press, Colorado.

Wilson-Barnet, J. (1978) 'Patients' emotional responses to barium X-ray', *Journal of Advanced Nursing*, **3**, 37–46.

Wilson-Barnet, J. (1989) 'Patient Teaching', in Macleod-Clark, J. and Hockey, L. *Further Research for Nursing*, Churchill Livingstone, Edinburgh.

Chapter 5

Facilitating therapeutic nursing and independent practice

STEPHEN WRIGHT

If nursing is to be therapeutic, then nurses must be able to recognise the breadth and potential they have in such a role. At the same time, the need to work in organisations which enable them to nurse therapeutically is paramount. Nightingale (1869) considered nursing as 'putting the patient in the best condition for nature to act'. How can nurses be put in a condition whereby nursing can act? Just as there are responsibilities laid at the feet of each nurse constantly to re-examine and improve the mode of her individual practice, so there is a need to examine the 'milieu' in which the nurse works.

THE INDIVIDUAL, THE ORGANISATION AND THERAPEUTIC NURSING

The UKCC (1984) has provided a code of conduct which maps out the nurse's role towards maintaining and developing standards of practise. Yet nursing which aspires to therapeutic values needs more than the commitment of the individual; it also needs a supportive climate in which to practise. The two are inseparable.

Historically, when nursing has failed, the trend has invariably been to seek out the scapegoat. Identifying and dismissing the 'bad' nurses is seen as resolving the problem. However, as Martin (1984) succinctly points out, 'Individual psychopathology may have a part, but the issues are both broader and deeper. They are broader in the sense that much turns on the attitudes of society to its weakest members [i.e.

the ill and vulnerable]. They are deeper in that what may occur is a perversion both of individual motives and of social institutions.' Thus, to facilitate therapeutic nursing it is necessary to look at what nurses believe about and do in nursing (the 'individual motives') but also the context (the 'social institutions', be they health care systems, hospital or nursing organisations) in which nursing is carried out.

Martin (1984) who surveyed over 30 major government and health authority enquiries into situations where health care had failed suggests that a number of key factors are significant:

1. The values which nurses hold depend not just upon those acquired while being socialised into nursing, but also those brought in from the wider culture in which they are raised.
2. The quality of leadership of the team in which nurses work.
3. The knowledge base which nurses and colleagues possess for practice, and the extent to which this is developed.
4. The resources available (funding for salaries, equipment, staffing levels etc.) to carry out nursing.
5. The degree to which nurses, and patients, are involved in the decision-making process on matters affecting care.
6. The facilities available for nursing practice e.g. buildings and design of the working environment.

A more recent report commissioned by the government of the day, and for very different motives, sought to explain the exodus of nurses from nursing (Price Waterhouse 1988). Interestingly, much of their findings mirrored the work of Martin (1984) and of the American 'Magnet' study (McLure et al., 1983). Fears related to demographic changes have led many to wonder where the nurses of the future will be recruited from (UKCC 1986). Yet even a changing structure of the population could not explain the difficulties of recruiting and retaining nurses. What had gone so terribly wrong with a profession, in which the attrition rate was so great, that nursing was having to reproduce itself every ten years, simply to keep enough nurses working 'at the bedside' with patients? (RCN 1986). The Price Waterhouse (1988) report pointed to a number of key areas of dissatisfaction, which can be summarised thus:

1. inadequate pay;
2. lack of support, and involvement in the decision-making

process, on the part of managers;
3. feeling undervalued at work, with little attention given to personal and professional development;
4. feeling unable to carry out nursing the way that it should be done.

While the loss of nurses from nursing is influenced by matters of pay and conditions, of equal if not greater importance to the nurse is the sense of personal worth and of 'doing a good job'. Indeed, an air of 'martyrdom' seems to pervade many avenues of nursing, as nurses continue to practise and struggle to maintain standards in spite of poor conditions of work and salary. While pay remains a factor in recruiting and retaining nurses (and the clinical regrading exercise began in 1988 sought to improve remuneration for clinical nurses), there are also a number of other key factors at work which must be considered. Even if clinical nurses achieve remarkable improvements in pay, the effects upon the loss of nurses from nursing is uncertain. Nurses will continue to leave nursing (or be discouraged from entering it) while they feel that the climate for practice is absent. For nurses to take on their therapeutic role requires more than just attention to financial rewards, they also demand the facility to place themselves in the best conditions for nursing to act.

THE CONDITIONS FOR THERAPEUTIC NURSING

From the above discussion, a number of significant factors can be identified which govern nursing practice. These factors not only determine whether nurses come into and remain in practice, but whether features prevail which enable them to develop that practice into something which moves beyond 'getting through the work' (Clark 1976). For nursing practice to become holistic, healing and humane, i.e. therapeutic, it requires a fertile ground in which to grow.

The nurse: commitment and values

Becoming and remaining a therapeutic nurse demands a (nursing) lifetime of commitment from each individual nurse. In moving from 'novice to expert' and becoming a 'connoisseur' of nursing (Benner 1984), the time is filled with the acquisition of new kinds of knowledge and skills and the testing of old ones. To some degree, the organisation has a commitment to develop nursing and nurses, but this does not abrogate the responsibility of each nurse to become expert by their own efforts. Keeping up to date through reading books and journals, and attending workshops, courses and conferences when possible are one side of the bargain which each nurse makes with the organisation in which he or she works.

However, if each nurse takes on the commitment towards expertise and excellence, then this raises a further question – to what end is this effort being applied? To suggest that each nurse should work for high standards of practice is simplistic unless the nature of that practice and the values which underpin it are explored and defined. In order to practise therapeutically, each nurse has to have a very clear vision of what nursing is – a healing art and science in its own right. Such nurses share positive values about all human beings – regardless of age, race, beliefs or sexuality. Elder (1977) believes that those who enter positions of caring for others must have 'a belief in the species, which is an integral part of the will to survive, and therefore a belief in life' which presupposes 'an acceptance of the doctrine that all individuals count and have a right to a full life'.

Therapeutic nurses must have taken on board such values about people. As such they will not countenance alternative approaches which at best tend to reduce patients to what the Briggs Report (1972) called 'the production line of care'. Patients are divided into a series of tasks to be completed, carried out by varying levels of staff according to status and experience, and no-one is left to care for the patient as a whole. The Ombudsman's Reports (1985 et seq.) alone testify to the many problems this brings for patients as they come to feel isolated and ignored in the hands of those who are ostensibly there to care for them. Hall (1969) regards such nursing as having declined beneath the level of professionalism and derides it as having become a 'trade'. Beyond this lie the extremes of the 'total institution' (Goffman 1961) where patients become mere dehumanised objects peripheral to nursing activity. In such places, graphically summarised in Martin's (1984) survey, the reductionist approach achieves its nadir. Nursing becomes the antithesis of therapeutic caring. The needs of individual human beings are ignored as the nursing system strives to create a routinised and ritualised approach to 'care' which preserves the status quo. The system is served, but not the patient.

The therapeutic nurse recognises not only the value of each person, but also that of nursing. To suggest that nursing is valuable may seem like a statement of the obvious. However, the question has to be asked as to *what kind* of nursing is valuable. For many nurses, there is still a tendency to dismiss some elements of their practice as 'basic' or 'menial'. Instrumental skills are deemed to be more important and have greater status attached to them. Such nurses, in Oakley's (1984) view have come to see themselves in the narcissistic mirror offered by medicine. Thus 'clever', 'skilled', 'real' nursing is usually closely associated with medical 'cure', with acute illness and a high degree of medical-technological intervention. The therapeutic nurse does not entirely reject such roles, for such instrumental activities are indeed a part of nursing support, but only a part. They are peripheral to the core of nursing and indeed might be considered valueless unless they are combined with certain other elements. Otherwise the nurse seen in the narcissistic mirror is a medical helper, a doctor's handmaiden or biological plumber's mate – anything but a nurse.

Therapeutic nursing may include many medico-technical or 'instrumental' skills, but at its heart lies the 'expressive' skills. It is the latter which the patient often sees as 'real' nursing, and about which he or she complains most bitterly when it fails (e.g. Ombudsman's Reports 1985 et seq.). These expressive skills include the ability to 'be with' the patient – sharing plans of care, teaching, comforting, informing. The therapeutic nurse works as a partner with the patient and acts as advocate when the patient is unwilling or unable to participate in choices about care. Campbell (1984) sees the nurse as expressing a form of 'moderated love' by acting as a form of 'companion' to the patient who seeks to share care with the patient, rather than imposing nursing upon him or her. These expressive skills lie at the very centre of nursing, and are part of the way in which therapeutic nurses are seen to act out their values. For them there is no such thing as 'basic' nursing. Helping an elderly man to use the washbasin again successfully, comforting the distressed child at night, relieving the pain of the post-operative patient where the drug is but a small part of the therapy –

these are tasks which some have dismissed as menial and therefore the territory of the nursing auxiliary or support worker. Yet these activities, and others like them, are the 'high touch' skills of nursing without which, the 'high tech' skills have little meaning. Without them, the patient may be treated but is not healed and feels alone and abandoned as a person.

The therapeutic nurse has a very clear idea of what constitutes nursing, and recognises that those acts often dismissed as basic, are actually complex, intricate and value elements in their own right. Without them, the essence of nursing is lost. It is nursing of a sort, but it is not therapeutic nursing. The challenge is to combine both facets, the instrumental and the expressive, into a healing whole which serves the patient. When nurses succeed in this they have come to terms with the value of nursing, and created a unique form of professionalism. If the functional, reductionist and institutional approach is the nadir of nursing, then its zenith is the therapeutic nurse.

The nurse as a change agent

Much of health care and particularly nursing is still organised along hierarchical and bureaucratic lines. To work professionally in such a system may in some way be seen as a contradiction in terms. The nurse may seek to exercise professional autonomy and make decisions about patient care (and indeed the organisation may seem to be encouraging him or her, at least superficially, to do so). Yet at the same time the nurse receives conflicting signals as others endeavour to exercise control over nursing practice such as doctors, senior nurses, finance directors, supplies officers and so on.

The struggle between the twin poles of professionalism and bureaucracy is mirrored in that between the holistic, therapeutic approach in nursing, and that which is reductionist and functional (e.g. the task-centred approach to care). To work successfully in such a climate demands considerable skills of nurses, for they must seek to change the nature of the organisation, or at least to neutralise its effects so that they can concentrate on therapeutic practice. Amongst these skills must be those of change agency.

Nursing has tended to experience a power-coercive approach to change in health care. Policies determined at

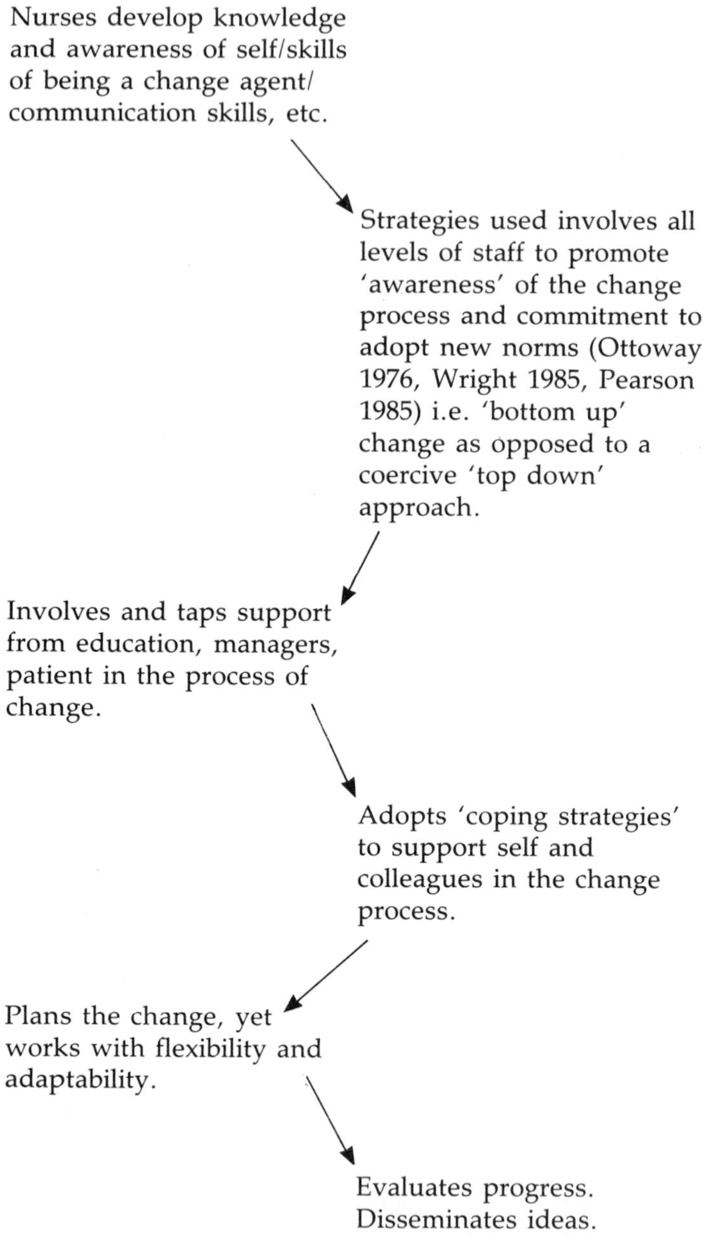

Nurses develop knowledge
and awareness of self/skills
of being a change agent/
communication skills, etc.

Strategies used involves all
levels of staff to promote
'awareness' of the change
process and commitment to
adopt new norms (Ottoway
1976, Wright 1985, Pearson
1985) i.e. 'bottom up'
change as opposed to a
coercive 'top down'
approach.

Involves and taps support
from education, managers,
patient in the process of
change.

Adopts 'coping strategies'
to support self and
colleagues in the change
process.

Plans the change, yet
works with flexibility and
adaptability.

Evaluates progress.
Disseminates ideas.

Figure 5.1 Elements of a change strategy.

higher levels are passed down through the hierarchy, with the nurse expected to put them into practice (Keyser 1989). This top-down approach is flawed. It leads to resistance and possibly ultimate failure of the proposed changes, because the nurses at the clinical level may not feel committed to or 'own' the new norms. Alternatives such as the normative-re-educative style ('bottom up') of change enables nurses actively to participate as change agents in their own practice, and is argued to be more successful (Pearson 1985, Wright 1989a).

All nurses are change agents. It may be at the level of helping a patient to adapt to a different lifestyle or educating for self care, or teaching students and colleagues to achieve mastery of nursing. In a grander sphere, it may be that they act to influence decisions in their health organisation, or their professional associations.

Perhaps nurses know 'what' needs changing, but it seems that they are less certain in the knowledge of 'how' to change. Many authors have recently argued for a planned approach to change (Pearson 1985, Turrill 1985, Pearson and Vaughan 1986, Salvage 1988, and Wright 1989a) and particularly for the development of the skills of nurses as change agents. A full discussion of change agency and strategies is beyond the scope of this chapter, but from the work of the authors cited above, a few key points can be suggested.

Figure 5.1 shows a few of the key features in a successful change strategy. However small or grand, the approach to change needs to be as planned and systematic as possible. Therapeutic nurses recognise their role as change agents, whether this involves working with individual patients, with larger groups or in much more wide-ranging activities. The implications for nurses recognising and making a greater use of their role are enormous. Nurses can not only help to produce an organisational climate where change is accepted as a way of life; they can also transport the effects way beyond the boundaries of the work place. There are over half a million nurses in the UK. If a majority, if not all, were to become self-aware, knowledgeable, skilled change agents, then the implications not just for nurses, or of health care but of society as a whole are enormous.

Providing the knowledge base

Having a knowledge of nursing and its value, and knowing

how to work in it as a change agent, are essential to the role of the therapeutic nurse. While to some degree each nurse has an obligation to attend to their own development, there is also an obligation on the part of the organisation in which he or she works. Nursing development units, such as those in Oxford and Tameside, have shown how the development of nursing is intimately linked to the development of nurses (Salvage 1989, Punton 1989, Bamber et al. 1989).

Developing nursing and nurses is, however, not the exclusive province of nursing development units, nor can it be abrogated to the school of nursing as its responsibility. It is also the province of the service sector in which the nurse works. The reputation of the latter in offering further education to nurses has initially been poor (Price Waterhouse 1988, RCN 1986). In a hard-pressed and often under-resourced service, an ethos has tended to develop that funding and time off for nurses cannot be afforded. However, the argument can be developed that the service cannot afford not to. High quality nursing needs high quality nurses. An investment in nurses in terms of time and money for their development is therefore an investment in the quality of patient care. There is some evidence to suggest that there is now increasing pressure within the general management of the NHS, for example, to address this issue (Department of Health 1989). Objectives suggested to managers to meet the needs of the service are now incorporating elements which encourage awareness (and meet objectives) of the needs of the staff.

The Price Waterhouse Report (1988) illustrated how nurses feelings about being valued by the organisation (in terms of being encouraged to develop) is strongly linked to recruitment and retention rates. However, it seems that large parts of health care have yet fully to accept this notion, although the benefits to both nursing and the organisation are clear. Therapeutic nursing can grow when the organisation supports it, and the development needs of nurses are thus satisfied. When nurses are developed, they feel more valued and reduce costs attributed to high staff turnover, sickness and absenteeism (Dean 1986).

The organisation can provide on-site development, or may tap the resources of local colleges and universities, or encourage participation in the enormous range of courses and workshops provided for nurses. Pearson (1988) and Purdy et al. (1988) have illustrated the direction such nursing developments should take – focusing on communication skills, assertiveness, self-awareness, research skills, complementary therapies etc., which assist nurses in the move along the trajectory from 'novice to expert' (Benner 1984). Recognising the financial difficulties which many settings experience, Purdy and Wright (1988) have suggested ways in which the organisation can generate income to enhance the limited funds which might otherwise be available.

The facilitation of therapeutic nursing does not, therefore, rely only on the personal commitment to development by the nurse. It also requires a whole-hearted commitment by the organisation to support the nurse. It is in their mutual interest to do so. Every setting should be a nursing development unit.

The organisational aspects

The development and support of therapeutic nursing requires a particular organisational climate. It is characterised by being non-hierarchical and allowing nurses to be involved in the decision-making process (McLure et al. 1983). Managers tend to have an open and supportive style and demonstrate qualities of leadership with which the staff feel at ease, free to develop, to criticise, to change and to ask questions. At ward level, this style of leadership is crucial for the ward sister (Pembrey 1980, Ogier 1981) whose behaviour is so crucial to the generation of a therapeutic nursing climate.

Sparrow (1986) has illustrated how the ward sister/charge nurse role shifts from being autocratic controller of the nursing staff, to supporter, teacher and encourager of nursing colleagues. Individual nurses, meanwhile, assume a greater autonomy and accountability for their practice over a limited case-load of patients resulting in the practice of primary nursing.

This management style and the squashing of the hierarchy where care is devolved to individual nurses is essential to liberate them to practise therapeutically. It is a management style which permits methods of organising care which can put nurses in a position where they can develop the 'partnership' relationship with patients. Many traditional approaches such as task allocation (Merchant 1985) and team nursing (Waters 1985) have tended to reduce nursing to a functional, reductionist approach. Patients become a series of tasks to be performed by varying nurses according to skill and status (aptly illustrated in Pearson and Vaughan 1986). The most senior nurse sits at the pinnacle carrying out the 'important' tasks (e.g. the ward sister and the doctor's 'round'), while other activities are delegated down, with the most junior dealing with the most 'menial'. Thinking about and organising care in the primary nursing (Pearson 1988, Wright 1989) approach is a radical shift away from these ideas. An individual (registered) nurse is accountable for the assessing, planning, implementing and evaluating of the care of a limited case-load of patients from admission through to discharge.

The development of primary nursing is highly complex and contentious, but it seems to be an approach which puts nurses in a position where they can act therapeutically. Nursing in this fashion requires a considerable degree of understanding between nurse and patient. Primary nursing facilitates this by enabling the nurse to work as a partner with the patient. The nurse gets involved. Methods such as task allocation limit nurse-patient involvement, and indeed, it has been argued, are actually used to prevent it, so that the nurse can cope more easily with the anxiety of nursing (Menzies 1961).

If task allocation became a defence mechanism to protect nurses in the fraught world of their practice, then primary nursing, which involves the nurse with the patient much more intimately, requires other methods to protect the nurse. The morality of unleashing nurses into this type of relationship with patients is questionable, if it is not concurrently backed up with a personal and managerial commitment to develop the nurse and the climate in which the nurse works. If the defensive props of tasks are removed, what is put in their place so that the nurse is not physically and psychologically exhausted by the work?

There appear to be two key areas for consideration. The first relates to the commitment to develop the nurse (referred to in 'Providing the knowledge base' above). The second relates to the creating of support mechanisms for nurses. Purdy et al. (1988) identified examples of these in their nursing development unit:

1. The formation of on-site peer groups and forums for mutual support.

2. Setting up a support team (consisting of the nurse manager, consultant nurse and nurse specialists) to provide counselling, development and clinical expertise.
3. Involving clinical nurses in quality assurance methods (patients are also included in this strategy), ward audits, standard setting, staff appraisal and appointments, budget management and so on.
4. Reviewing and revising skill mixes to enable primary nursing to develop and review the work of the support roles (e.g. ward clerks).
5. Setting up an extensive staff development and research programme involving all grades of staff and planned on a continuous basis.
6. Facilitating 'quality circles' (Christie 1986) which enable problem solving on day-to-day working practices and difficulties to be devolved to ward level.
7. Applying maximum resources to improving the working environment (e.g. furnishings, decorating, facilities) or to equipment needed to facilitate nursing practice (e.g. modern beds, revised nursing documentation etc.).

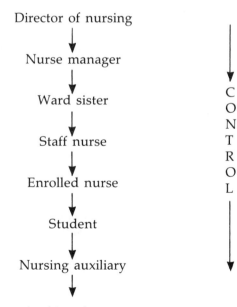

Figure 5.2 A typical nursing hierarchy.

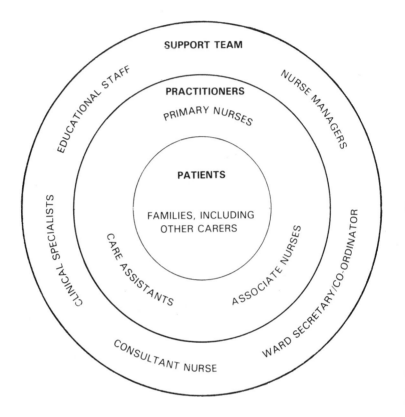

Figure 5.3 An organisational structure supportive of therapeutic nursing.

The general aims of these and other principles suggested is to devolve the maximum power, control and accountability of nursing to those nurses who are in practice, and enabling them to develop their roles at minimal risk to themselves and their patients. Thus, the organisational structure needed to support therapeutic nursing has to be reviewed from the traditional mode to a structure such as that shown in figure 5.3. For nurses to act therapeutically, they need not only a method of organising care to do so, but a supportive organisational structure which facilitates them.

BOUNDARIES OF NURSING?

A shift in nursing practice which emphasises the healing role of the nurse, and additionally assumes a degree of independent practice, has significant implications for inter-disciplinary relationships as well as for patients and relatives. MacDonald (1988) and Bowers (1988) have suggested numerous conflicts for nurses who develop primary nursing. Expectations of patients, relatives and members of the multi-disciplinary team may be in conflict with the traditional role of the nurse. Young et al. (1988) and Strong and Robinson (1988) suggest there may be worries for managers about containing the costs of nursing, or even, of keeping it firmly under control in the widest sense. In developing their role, nurses disrupt the status quo of established 'role sets' and 'role expectations' (Argyle 1978).

The development of nurses – their awareness of themselves, of the organisation, and of their capacity as change agents, is essential in the move towards therapeutic nursing. The changeover of roles puts nurses on a collision course with the establishment and ultimately they may need all the skills at their disposal to minimise the shock of the repercussions which occur in other roles.

Many colleagues may be willing supporters of nurses in their change of role, while others may resist, become hostile or obstructive, or actively seek to destroy nursing innovation (Salvage 1985). The term 'multi-disciplinary team' conjures up an image of mutual respect and authority within the team, each member being committed to the benefit of the patient. The reality may be somewhat different, particularly for nurses (predominantly female) who must deal with (predominantly male) doctors. Medical authority remains the most potent of all and nurses must often indulge in the 'doctor-nurse game' (Stein 1978) to achieve their goals in patient care without threatening the dominant position of the doctor.

While nurses must work with a variety of disciplines, there has been relatively little work undertaken on evaluating multi-disciplinary teams. Does the ideal of a team of equals, with each contributing to the patient's needs according to skills (rather than one discipline ruling the others) work in reality?

McFarlane (1980) claims that the narrow disease orientation of the NHS, coupled with undue emphasis on medical function, have served to concentrate attention on the role of the doctor and minimise the contribution and potential of other health workers. The extent to which doctors will relinquish their traditionally dominant role in the team is debatable. While some doctors appear to accept the development of the therapeutic role of the nurse others (Rastan 1989) have shown a marked hostility and have contributed to a reversal of nursing innovation (Naish 1989).

Recognising the potential for conflict is an important aspect of the role of the therapeutic nurse, for it will occur in varying degrees with all levels of the multi-disciplinary team. Awareness of these difficulties and the possibilities of managing them, can contribute significantly to the skills of the therapeutic nurse in defusing them. In time, if the therapeutic role of the nurse survives and spreads, then a corresponding adjustment of role perceptions by those in other disciplines must ensue. It will be the generations of nurses in the future who will be in a position to judge the success or failure of the role of therapeutic nurses.

SUMMARY

The success, or otherwise, of the therapeutic role of the nurse will be determined not only by nurses themselves, but also the nature of the organisation in which they work and the degree of support they receive from their colleagues. Many of the obstacles and potential conflicts can be overcome by examining the way each nurse is prepared and what each setting can do to support nurses in the development of their practice. Financial rewards, re-examining values, education, learning change agency, improving the environment, reorganising patterns of care and creating support structures – these are some of the key features in enabling therapeutic nursing to happen. Such nurses are out on the boundaries of professional practice. They are testing the territory of traditional practices. They cannot be left to take such risks alone.

REFERENCES

Argyle, M. (1978) *The Psychology of Interpersonal Behaviour*, Penguin, Harmondsworth.

Bamber, T., Johnson, M.L., Purdy, E. and Wright, S. (1989) 'The Tameside experience', *Nursing Standard*, **22**(3) 26.

Benner, P. (1984), *From Novice to Expert*, Addison-Wesley, London.

Bowers, L. (1988) 'The significance of primary nursing', *Journal of Advanced Nursing*, **14** 13–19.

Briggs, et al. (1972) *Report of the Committee on Nursing* (Chairman: Professor Asa U. Briggs), HMSO/DHSS, London.

Campbell, A.V. (1984), *Moderated Love*, SPCK, London.

Christie, H. (1986) 'Quality circles – staff ideas are your richest resource', *Health Service Options*, p. 17.

Clark, M. (1978) 'Getting through the work', in Dingwall, R. and McIntosh, J. (eds.) *Readings in the Sociology of Nursing*, Churchill Livingstone, Edinburgh.

Dean, D. (1986) *Manpower Solutions*, Schutari Publication, London.

Department of Health (Nursing Division) (1989) *A Strategy for Nursing*, London.

Elder, G. (1977) *The Alienated – Growing Old Today*, Writers' and Readers' Publishers' Co-operative, London.

Goffman, I. (1961) *Asylums*, Penguin, Harmondsworth.

Hall, L.E. (1969) 'The Loeb Centre for Nursing and Rehabilitation', *International Journal of Nursing Studies*, **6** 82–3.

Keyser, D. (1989) Meeting the challenge: strategies for implementing change in Wright, S. (ed.) *Changing Nursing Practice*, Edward Arnold, London.

MacDonald, M. (1988) 'Primary nursing: is it worth it?' *Journal of Advanced Nursing*, **13** 797–806.

Martin, J.P. (1984) *Hospitals in Trouble*, Basil Blackwell, Oxford.

McFarlane, J.K. (1980) *Multi-disciplinary Clinical Teams*, Kings Fund, London.

McLure, M.L., Poulin, M.A., Sorie, M.D. and Wandelt, M.A. (1983) *Magnet Hospitals – Attraction and Retention of Professional Nurses*, American Academy of Nursing, Kansas City.

Menzies, I. (1961) 'The functioning of social systems as a defence against anxiety', reprinted in Menzies-Lyth, I. (1988) *Containing Anxiety in Institutions*, Free Association Books, London.

Merchant, I. (1985) 'Why task allocation?', *Nursing Practice*, **1**(2), 67–71.

Naish, J. (1989) 'Picking up the pieces' *Nursing Standard*, **25**(3), 13.

Nightingale, F. (1859) *Notes on Nursing* (Republished 1980), Churchill Livingstone, Edinburgh.

Oakley, A. (1984) 'The importance of being a nurse', *Nursing Times*, **80**(50), 24–7.

Ogier, M. (1981) *An Ideal Sister*, Royal College of Nursing, London.

Reports of the Parliamentary Liaison Officer (Ombudsman) for the Health Service (1985 et seq.) Department of Health, London.

Ottoway, R.N. (1976) 'A change strategy to implement new norms, new styles and new environment in the work organisation', *Personnel Review*, **5**(1), 13–18.

Pearson, A. (1985) 'The effects of introducing new norms in a nursing unit: an analysis of the process of change', Unpublished PhD Thesis,

Goldsmiths College, University of London.

Pearson, A. (ed.) (1988) *Primary Nursing*, Croom Helm, London.

Pearson, A. and Vaughan, B. (1986) *Nursing Models for Practice*, Heinemann, London.

Pembrey, S. (1980) *The Ward Sister – Key to Nursing*, Royal College of Nursing, London.

Price Waterhouse (1988) *Nurse Retention and Recruitment*, Price Waterhouse, London.

Punton, S. (1989) 'The Oxford Experience', *Nursing Standard* **22**(3), 271–8.

Purdy, E. and Wright, S.G. (1988), 'If I were a rich nurse', in *Nursing Times* **84**(41), 36–8.

Purdy, E., Wright, S.G. and Johnson, M.L. (1988) 'Change for the better', *Nursing Times*, **84**(38), 34–6.

Rastan, C. (1989) 'Angels who are more than guardians', *The Independent*, June 26th.

Royal College of Nursing (1986) *The Education of Nurses: a New Dispensation*, Royal College of Nursing, London.

Salvage, J. (1985) *The Politics of Nursing*, Heinemann Publishing Group Ltd., Oxford.

Salvage, J. (1988) 'Facilitating model-based nursing', unpublished paper, Nursing Models Conference, Gateshead.

Salvage, J. (1989) Nursing development units, *Nursing Standard*, **22**(3), 25.

Sparrow, S. (1986) 'Primary nursing' *Nursing Practice* **1**(3), 142–7.

Stein, L. (1978) 'The doctor-nurse game', in Dingwall, R. and MacIntosh, J. (eds) (1978) *Readings in the Sociology of Nursing*, Churchill Livingstone, Edinburgh.

Strong, P. and Robinson, J. (1988) *New Model Management: Griffiths and the NHS*, Nursing Policy Studies, University of Warwick, Warwick.

Turrill, T. (1988) *Change and Innovation: A Challenge for the NHS*, Management Series 10, Institute of Health Service Management, London.

United Kingdom Central Council for Nursing, Midwifery and Health Visitors (1984) *Code of Professional Conduct for the Nurse, Midwife and Health Visitor*, UKCC, London.

United Kingdom Central Council for Nursing, Midwifery and Health Visiting (1986) *Project 2000*, UKCC, London.

Waters, K. (1985), 'Team nursing' *Nursing Practice* **1**(1), 7–15.

Wright, S.G. (1985) 'Change in nursing: the application of change theory to practice', *Nursing Practice*, **1**(2), 85–91.

Wright, S.G. (1989a) *Changing Nursing Practice*, Edward Arnold, London.

Wright, S.G. (1989b) *My Nurse: My Patient – Primary Nursing in Practice*, Scutari, London.

Young, J.P., Giovanetti, P., Lewison, D. and Thoms, M.L. (1981) *Factors Affecting Nurse Staffing in Acute Care Hospitals: a Review and Critique of the Literature (DHEW Publication No. HRP0801801)*, Department of Health Education and Welfare, Hyattsville.

Chapter 6

Tailoring research for advanced nursing practice

JILLIAN MACGUIRE

'Kitson (1986) has appealed for a methodology to validate the hitherto intangible and elusive qualities of caring. "Intuition and experience" are daily used to justify action, but since a hit-and-miss attitude is morally and professionally indefensible where persons of value are concerned, this mystique of the nurse demands to be brought to consciousness and clarity, and a place in the research base and methodology of practice. Once achieved not only can its essence be communicated and taught but its influence may *inform* caring by providing guidelines for the selection of methods and a frame of reference for prescriptive choices for action and interaction . . . .

Plaxy-Anita Muetzel, 1988

INTRODUCTION

This chapter looks in a broad way at the contribution of research to nursing practice and, more specifically, at how therapeutic nursing might be advanced through research. Key questions to address are whether the study of nursing practice demands the use of particular research methodologies, what these might be and whether resources for such research are likely to be restricted because of the very methodologies advocated. Finally consideration is given to some of the difficulties associated with isolating what might be regarded as nursing outputs and with the adoption of research-based knowledge into clinical practice.

Though there is now an extensive body of work that may be labelled nursing research and a growing number of nurses, as well as people from other disciplines, are directly engaged in research activity, it is doubtful if nursing can, as yet, sustain the claim to being a research-based profession. In part, this is because not all nurses engaged in patient care fully accept the arguments for research-based practice. Many do not feel that research necessarily has relevance to their own work and fail to seek a role for themselves in the development of practice through research. Research, for a variety of reasons, has not always addressed the concerns of clinical nurses and frequently does not produce the kind of reliable guide to practice that practitioners require. The research process is clouded in mystery and the results are sometimes couched in impenetrable language.

Nursing research as an identifiable and separate discipline has a relatively short history. That of research into practice is even briefer (Hunt 1987). Since therapeutic nursing is only on the edge of the consciousness of the profession it might be anticipated that relevant research into its practice is limited. This may be, as McMahon (1989) suggests, because it is still a character in search of an author and, therefore, lacks an accepted definition and partly because it is difficult to see how the process and outcomes of such practice might be researched.

Nursing research cannot so far lay claim to the invention of any methodology peculiar to itself. Instead it draws on a wide range of methodologies from other disciplines; an eclectic approach which offers a wealth of possibilities but no single, definitive pathway. In principle, the choice depends on the proclivities of the researcher and the nature of the research question. In practice things are not that simple.

The main distinction is between quantitative methodologies, which have their origins in the natural sciences and are concerned with proof and prediction, and qualitative methodologies which have been developed in the social sciences and are concerned with the knowledge, understanding and perceptions people have of their worlds and how this affects their actions. The difference is not just one of methods of investigation but of philosophical dispute about the nature of knowledge, the purpose of research and the relationship between investigator and subject.

It is tempting to try to resolve the qualitative/quantitative debate by arguing that 'the problem dictates the method of investigation' (Trow quoted in Lathlean and Farnish 1984) but this apparently simple solution obscures two associated difficulties. The first is that the conceptualisation of research as a 'problem-solving activity' suggests that there is a 'problem' and that the problem has been properly identified, a potential pitfall identified by Menzies (1966) in her work on student nurses. The second is that it implies that there must be an answer that can underpin policy initiatives and practice guidelines. Moreover, it appears to deny the converse of the proposition which is that a particular methodological approach may itself be used to determine the research question. This may result in the formulation of inappropriate questions and misguided research effort.

What is it that leads both practitioners and researchers to question the applicability of available methodologies? Firstly, there is the pervading myth of the 'uniqueness' of nursing which, while often not brought into the open in discussions about methodology, underpins the search for a 'nursing' research methodology. Secondly, there is a defensiveness which seeks to protect nursing research from criticism by incorporating and misappropriating other methodologies. 'Ethnonursing research' is an example of this tendency. Workers in the nursing field ought to be able to take an ethnomethodological approach without needing to create a specifically *nursing* version. There is a very real danger that this process may lead to nurse researchers being inadequately prepared in the rigours of the particular methodology and thus to using it in ways which do not stand comparison with the work of the experts in the discipline. Thirdly, there is a propensity to jump on the latest methodological bandwagon in order to demonstrate that nursing research is out there in the forefront. Fourthly, the view that nursing is both art and science and can, therefore, be studied neither as pure science nor pure art without misrepresentation. This standpoint is sometimes used to devalue all research and as an excuse for not subjecting practice to enquiry.

Fifthly, and this must be seriously considered, there is the argument that nursing is a *practice* discipline and as such requires that research be contextual, related to and carried out in the workplace whether this be home, hospice or hospital. 'The centrality of practice to nursing mandates a bond between nursing research . . . and nursing practice' (Jennings and Rogers 1988). This suggests that one of the characteristics of nursing research is that it should be small-scale and practice-related and, therefore, may not be generalisable beyond the immediate situation. Finally, there is the idea that research should be focused primarily on the interaction between nurse and patient because this relationship mediates all nursing activity. Integral to such a view is the idea of the primacy for nursing research of the viewpoints, perceptions, understandings and intentions of the participants.

It is suggested that available methodologies do not enable us to understand patients as actors and initiators of their own strategies for dealing with illness, pain, discomfort or stress or to grasp the meanings that they attribute to the actions of nurses. Nor do they help to make clear what it is that nurses and nursing are about; the meaning of caring or nurturing or the essentially therapeutic nature of nursing interventions.

McMahon (1989) has defined therapeutic nursing as 'nursing that *deliberately* has beneficial outcomes for patients'. This definition suggests not only that all nursing activities should be planned but that the only legitimate activities are those which can be shown to have a positive effect for patients. This, indeed, would constitute research-based practice.

Can therapeutic nursing be defined and practised in ways that make it possible to research? What evidence is there that nurses and researchers are interested in this concept of nursing? Are there genuine problems about methodology or are the difficulties more to do with ethics, access, training and resources? How are we to look at outcomes for patients and how are we to know that they are beneficial?

FUNDING, ACCESS AND ETHICAL COMMITTEE APPROVAL

Muetzel (1988) has stated that nurse researchers have neglected certain areas of research and certain forms of research in favour of the 'scientific' methods associated with medical research. We need first to ask whether this contention is true and secondly why this should have happened. While it may be fashionable to talk about the art and science of nursing, nursing as it has entered into the academic arena in the UK has tended to be associated with existing faculties whether of biological sciences, social sciences, medicine or education. Both the social sciences and education, as academic disciplines, have had to make their own bids for academic and scientific recognition. We should not, therefore, be surprised if the research methodologies current in those departments have also tended to be adopted by nursing research. One strand lies in the search for academic respectability in general and in the bid for medical recognition in particular. Nursing research has from its origins had to assert itself as being something other than a handmaiden to medical research. Until recently professional relevance and clinical credibility have been seen as of lesser importance.

Medicine has developed a very powerful research design in the randomised cross-over clinical trial and there is an extensive literature on its development and use. The design should not be undervalued in nursing research nor denigrated because it is derived from medicine. It has been used effectively (Luker 1983) but may also be used inappropriately.

The social sciences have made great use of large-scale sample surveys based on carefully constructed and pre-tested questionnaires. A great deal of nursing research has drawn on this tradition. At the same time, much of this work has been criticised for being small scale, unrepresentative and thus not generalisable.

All research costs money; large-scale research requires large-scale financing. Even small-scale exploratory work requires money to employ appropriately qualified staff and additional cash for the running costs of a project. Universities are no longer willing or able to carry the hidden costs of research and grant applications to funding bodies have to take this into account. Nursing research, like all other research, is becoming more expensive at the same time as research funding from all sources is becoming more restricted. Emphasis on value for money and the ascendancy of policy-driven research must inevitably have some effect on the kinds of research project that ultimately secure funding. This is true for all areas of research and not just for nursing.

Nursing research can call on no separate, identifiable budgets at national, regional or local level within the structure of NHS financing nor is there specific funding within the university or educational sectors. There is no Nursing Research

Council. Nursing research has to compete directly with medical research for Department of Health funding or for funding from the Medical Research Council (MRC). If it is looking for money from other research councils, it has to bid with all comers. Bids there are unlikely to be successful unless collaborative work is proposed because the natural sources of funding for nursing research are perceived to be either the Department of Health or the MRC. Few nursing researchers to date have been successful in obtaining MRC funding.

The main financing of nursing research is through the Department of Health's directly managed projects. In 1988 about 7% of the £13.6 million spent under this heading went to programmes which are clearly identifiable as 'nursing research' in that they are about some aspect of the organisation of nursing, the recruitment and education of nurses or the delivery of nursing care. While it is not always possible to tell from the title the exact nature of the research approach adopted the emphasis would appear to be on large-scale survey research though other approaches are by no means excluded.

Major funding for nursing research from this source can only be obtained by adherence to the Rothschild principles. These require that the customer, which is the Department of Health, should commission such research. Proposals have to fall within the current priorities established by the Department of Health and to provide 'objective information for Ministers on ways of improving the efficiency and effectiveness of the HPSS and Social Security by promoting improvements in organisation, operation and administration' (DHSS 1989). Clinical nursing research may not have a high priority on these agendas and may be seen as a more narrowly professional matter for which funding should be sought elsewhere.

Small amounts of money are also available for research which does not have an identified customer. In addition post-graduate and post-doctoral awards are made by the Department of Health to support nursing research activities. These proposals too have to fall within stated priority areas though, in practice, there seems to be considerable flexibility. Finance for clinical work can be obtained. The strength of the research design rather than the specific theoretical or methodological approach is probably the major determinant of success.

Non-governmental research funding bodies and charitable organisations also support nursing research. They will also have their own priorities which are bound to be reflected in the nature of the projects they are prepared to finance. Research which is perceived as having immediate practical applicability or which addresses some major current concern is likely to be seen as more attractive than more theoretical work or, indeed, more basic work.

Professor Asa Briggs, as chairman of the Committee on Nursing, in advocating that nursing should become a research-based profession saw health authorities as having a major role to play a funding clinical research (HMSO 1972) and the Royal Commission on the National Health Service (HMSO 1979) advocated the creation of joint appointments linking clinical and research activity. Some authorities began to appoint nurse researchers but recent financial cutbacks have meant that many of these appointments have often been short-lived. Sometimes people appointed were required to be self-financing through the introduction of savings in the nursing budget while others were employed to provide nursing management information rather than to develop nursing practice through research. The creation and recognition of nursing development units may be a more viable way of securing clinical nursing research at local level. Researchers appointed to them may be less peripheral.

The development of clinical nursing research depends in part on the ease with which individuals can move between clinical and research settings and the degree of autonomy they are allowed in choosing what research to undertake. Increasing numbers of nurses are being funded by their employing authorities to register for higher degrees on a part-time basis. Most of such courses require students to prepare a research dissertation or to carry out small-scale research projects. Some of this work is clinically orientated and innovative but, inevitably, limited by the time constraints imposed. Courses currently being developed in research for practitioners place a high premium on tailoring teaching of research methodology to the practice concerns of the participants not all of whom are likely to be nurses. These innovations are productive in so far as they allow clinical nurses to get a grounding in research but restrictive if the research undertaken has to fit into the agenda of the employing authority or the researchers run into difficulties over ethical approval and access simply because of their dual status.

Funding for nursing research is closely tied up with questions of access and ethical committee approval. Those who control access and those who give ethical committee approval may also seek to influence research methodology and study design. The more nearly the research touches clinical issues and focuses on sensitive areas such as pain or patients' feelings about surgery, sexual behaviour or the perceived value of treatment regimens, the more likely it is that difficulties will be encountered in keeping these issues separate. Embargoes on funding and access can sometimes be issued from very high places leaving researchers with very little room in manoeuvre.

Pressure to adopt a quantitative rather than a qualitative approach and to employ an experimental research design frequently comes directly from the members of ethical committees. Medical researchers are themselves critical of the way in which ethical committees seek to control access and research design (Institute of Medical Ethics Bulletin 1989) but often ignore real ethical issues. These committees often sit without a proper brief or agreed criteria for accepting or rejecting proposals which come before them (West Birmingham CHC 1988).

Funding is often dependent on prior agreements about access and ethical committee approval. Nurses sometimes experience difficulties with ethical committees but rarely report on such problems in their research papers because of the understandable fear that any future research proposals might be in jeopardy were they to put their criticisms and experiences on record.

Some of the difficulty arises because the idea of nurses doing research at all is still unfamiliar, and partly because qualitative methods are not entirely understood within such committees which may only rarely include a sociologist or anthropologist. Criteria more applicable to experimental work are applied and proposals are inevitably seen to fall short. A few medical clinicians try to use their position on such committees to block access to *their* patients. In such a context nurse researchers may well feel that proposals which fit medical design canons and which do not concentrate on patients' experience of their treatment are more likely to succeed.

Clinical medical research is in part legitimated by the clinical position and therapeutic orientation of doctors. Nurses undertaking research are often recently qualified or hold marginal positions in the nursing hierarchy. As more clinical nursing research is undertaken by practitioners in clinical nursing career posts and as nursing is seen to have an independent therapeutic contribution it may become easier to get access to patients in medically dominated areas.

While such clinical nurse researchers employed in practice settings are in no way absolved from seeking ethical approval for their research and, indeed, have special responsibilities to their patients because of such a dual role, access to patients is legitimated by their clinical position. Also because they are participants in the clinical situation by right they may be able more readily to use qualitative approaches in their work and to undertake research in aspects of clinical work which have previously seemed too difficult or too dangerous.

Much of the more qualitative research is currently carried out by nurses in the course of their higher degree work. Because many of them go back into clinical, teaching or management posts rather than continuing in research this work is often not published and is, therefore, not developed by other researchers. A lot of valuable work lies buried in theses which practitioners and even researchers may never think to access.

CLINICAL NURSING RESEARCH

Pearson's (1988) prophetic statement that 'the future of practical, hands-on nursing obviously lies in the hands of clinical nurses – who need to assert the potential of nursing as a means of healing' is a good starting point for the consideration of the relationship between practice and research. One vehicle for asserting the value of nursing as healing is through research which demonstrates the efficacy of nursing intervention.

Clinical nursing covers a broad spectrum of nursing activity. Any part of that activity may be called into question, through research, in terms of the contribution it makes to the well-being of patients, to the recovery process, to rehabilitation and to the maintenance of health. It is not self-evident that *nursing* and *nurses* make a difference to outcomes for patients. Until relatively recently nurses have worked in a climate in which their work has been tacitly accepted at its face value. Both overtly and covertly the value of nursing is being brought into question. It is now becoming increasingly urgent to evaluate independent nursing interventions both as a means of describing the essential core of nursing work and as part of the justification of the continued employment of highly trained professionals in the care of patients.

The concepts of *independent* nursing intervention and of *healing* are both crucial in determining the direction of research into clinical nursing practice. In what sense can nursing be regarded as independent? And how may nursing be understood as healing? It is only when we are able to define these terms satisfactorily that it is possible to design and undertake research which will support or refute the proposition that independent nursing intervention promotes healing.

Hockey's (1989b) typology of nursing activities as consisting of autonomous, derived and delegated elements suggests we should focus on the interventions which are initiated as well as undertaken by nurses. This is the core of nurses' work. It is what nurses do which is not done by other people. Nursing has always found it difficult to describe this core. Goddard's (Nuffield Provincial Hospitals Trust 1954) choice of the term 'basic' to describe this element of nursing work has had a disastrous influence not only on nurses' perceptions of the value of their work but also on the way in which nursing is regarded by other professional groups. It has been suggested that the term was used as a shorthand for 'fundamental' or 'essential' and that it has been systematically misinterpreted over the last three decades by those who wish to use it to justify the horizontal division of nursing labour. Goddard demonstrated that basic nursing was undertaken by the least qualified and the lowest skilled. This observation might have sparked off a revolution in the delivery of nursing care but instead it has been and is used to justify the continued employment of unskilled labour in direct patient care. The competencies being outlined for the support worker suggests that this process will be extended yet again. As Robinson et al. (1989) put it: 'Debate about the role of support staff undoubtedly disguises debate about the future of nursing itself'. The substitution of the terms 'direct patient care' or 'hands-on care' for 'basic care' gets slightly closer to the heart of the matter but we still remain in the realms of an instrumental under-standing of nursing.

Smith (1988) has explored the relevance of the concept of emotional labour to nursing. Emotional labour is concerned with establishing and maintaining affective states; subjective feelings of comfort, security, well-being, safety and worth. Derived from a study of airline cabin staff by Hochschild (1985), this idea adds a new dimension to the analysis of the work of nursing. It is the 'how' rather than the 'what' of the activity that is highlighted. Superficially there may seem to be little in common between an intensive care ward and a jumbo jet. But aircraft, like hospitals, are 'institutions cradled in anxiety' (Revans 1962). Throughput of patients and passengers is high. Instrumentality predominates. Danger, crisis, failure and death are potentially overwhelming for all parties in the enterprise. Space is confined and the normal range of behaviour restricted. Intimacy with total strangers is not only allowed but legitimated. Nurses and cabin staff make use of sexual allure and plan on patient and passenger fantasies. Patients and passengers are dependent on others for survival. Key functions of both cabin staff and nurses are to create an atmosphere of normality. Homeliness is seen as an important aspect of both environments. Making the cabin seem like your own front room or the ward like your own back bedroom are believed to reduce the fear engendered by unfamiliarity. Staff are expected to offer reassurance as well as re-hydration, comfort as well as cuisine provençale, understanding as well as unguent. In each case the latter is the medium for conveying the message. The message, whether to passenger or patient, is that each is unique, important, valued and that the steward or nurse is concerned in a deeply personal way about their comfort, their anxieties and their needs. The emotional labour lies in the maintenance of states of well-being among passengers or patients. It is not window dressing or packaging though it may deteriorate into that if too great a demand is made of staff by the managers of emo-tional labour. It is not a by-product or unintended consequence of physical or intellectual activities. Emotional labour is the essential element which defines and differentiates. For nursing there is, perhaps, a higher goal in that nursing involves the use of self in an intentionally therapeutic way to create and maintain a sense of well-being among patients.

Patients judge nurses on their emotional style (Smith 1989). Their competence they take for granted. That this may, in some cases, turn out to be unwarranted makes it all the more important that the technical aspects of nurses' work should be rooted in research-based practice so that we do, indeed, act in such a way that we do the patient no harm. The value patients place on emotional work alerts us to the idea that they may not respond in expected ways to nursing care however technically excellent unless nurses get what Hochschild calls the 'deep acting' right. They must convey information, through actions rather than solely through words, about emotional care in order to facilitate other aspects of care. A nurse cannot '*make* a patient comfortable' and she certainly cannot bring about a change through the medium of words alone. She can only recognise discomfort, attend to a patient's wishes or needs, express her concern and then, with the patient, use technical skills to solve the problem that faces them both. You only have to read Victor Zorza's (1980) account of how a nurse in a hospice struggled to make his daughter Jane comfortable to understand just how difficult this is. Concentrating on the emotional labour of nursing does not mean that what we do at a technical level does not matter so long as we get the feeling right. The implication is that technical care, however excellent, may fall short of its therapeutic intent unless attention is paid to the emotional aspect of care.

It is a short step from the idea of well-being to that of healing. Healing is the restoration of the feeling of well-being, the replacement of comfort for discomfort, ease for disease, security for insecurity and, in the hymn writer J.S.B. Mansell's words, 'Trust for our trembling and hope for our fear' (English Hymnal No. 42).

CATEGORIES OF THERAPEUTIC NURSING

Most nursing care is not delivered and received via a continuous didactic relationship but through serial relationships. This raises questions about the level at which the 'nurse-patient relationship' may be held to exist in practice. This, in turn, raises questions about the very possibility of therapeutic nursing particularly where this is grounded in the therapeutic use of self.

Muetzel (1988) has argued that the adoption of primary nursing is a prerequisite for the practice of therapeutic nursing. Binnie (1987) has stated bluntly that nursing structures are in the main inimical to the introduction and support of primary nursing. On this basis therapeutic nursing is likely to be practised in very few places at present though the idea is gaining currency. Wharton and Pearson (1988) write that 'the complex, therapeutic role of both primary and associate nurse, rooted in close relationships and an environment for healing and growth hinges, we believe, on the hands of the nurse being used therapeutically in giving direct care'. If this sounds more like the prayer of St Theresa than a procedure manual it is because many such assertions are at the moment tentative hypotheses or propositions which are awaiting research. Where is the research evidence, for example, that the use of night sedation has fallen notably since the initiation of massage for sleeplessness? This may well be the experience of the nurses working in that particular situation but before such practices are taken up in other areas it is important to demonstrate the link between the two variables. The implication that it is the controlled experiment itself which destroys what it sets out to study and, therefore, fails to produce positive evidence should be strenuously resisted. At the same time it must be recognised that in social situations any intervention of any kind may bring about observable and even measurable change. The particular intervention may not be causally linked with the observed change as, for example, with the use of placebo drug therapy. The intervention may simply offer the opportunity for an exchange between nurse and patient and the therapeutic result may stem from the quality of that exchange. Such complicated issues have to be faced if we are not to introduce new practice on an inadequate footing.

Ersser (1988) has suggested five broad categories for describing the therapeutic approach to nursing. These are the nurse-patient relationship, creating a therapeutic environment, giving information, providing comfort and holistic health practices. McMahon (1989) has added a sixth, that of tested physical interventions. While a literature search using 'therapeutic nursing' may not yield much in the way of research-based references (Hockey 1989b), exploration of the component elements is more productive. A search using the CD Silver Platter v 1.5 search and retrieval system which covers journal articles from 1983 to 1989 yielded 86 references on comfort, 192 on touch of which 28 related specifically to therapeutic touch, 37 on empathy and 51 on therapeutics and nursing. A search using the Royal College of Nursing's in-house system yielded 1100 items on therapy, 148 items in response to the key-word 'therapeutic' of which, on inspection, 43 were relevant, though few were research-based, and 33 on comfort. There were, in addition, many research-based references on the therapeutic community in psychiatric care. 'Deliberative nursing', an American term in the same area of interest, produced only one item and that related to good chairmanship! McMahon's contention that the term 'therapeutic nursing' has yet to find an owner and a definition would seem to be borne out by its non-appearance in contents and key-word lists, yet there is ample evidence that these issues are being addressed and, to a limited extent, researched.

The DHSS *Handbook of Research and Development 1988* lists 852 recent publications by directors and project leaders and their staff. Of these 36 have nurses, nursing, health visitors, health visiting, midwives or midwifery in their title. None of these relate to 'therapeutic' issues in nursing as defined by McMahon. Of the remaining references there is one paper which explores the effect of the environment on the dependency of elderly people in residential homes (Netten 1988).

Bond and Bond (1982) used the Delphi technique to explore in a systematic way what nurses wanted to see researched. The rationale for this approach being that 'utilisation of research would be more likely to occur if the initial research had high social relevance'. Nearly half of the items (48%) related to nursing practice. While the term 'therapeutic nursing' does not appear, communication, the management of pain and the care of the terminally ill were ranked highly in terms of their importance for both nurses and patients. Determining methods of encouraging greater utilisation of research findings in nursing practice was high on the agenda but in terms of its value to nurses themselves, rather than to patients. This is an interesting perceptual difference suggesting that research is seen as having potential to improve the practice of nurses but not as a major contribution to the welfare of patients.

It is not the purpose of this chapter to present a bibliographic review of research on therapeutic nursing. It is sufficient to demonstrate that there is an emerging literature on this topic though much of it is not research-based. The material on touch is extensive and illustrates the use of a number of research methodologies. Classic experimental work was carried out on the importance of touch to baby monkeys (Harlow and Harlow 1966). That scientific or positivist methods have to be used in proofs of practice does not imply the denial of the uniqueness of the individual patient and the individual nurse. The randomised cross-over trial (Keller and Bzdek 1986) may well be the most appropriate research design for establishing the relative effectiveness of therapeutic touch in pain control while the understanding, use and value to the patient of therapeutic touch in a practice setting may best be explored through ethnographic methods. Touch, for example, may signify acceptance, inclusion and belonging. It may confirm feelings of self-worth or even bring about awareness of being in the world. These may be important benefits in their own right or may help people to be less aware or tuned-in to their pain. The relationship between the objective fact of pain and the subjective experience of the patient or use of touch and the subjective meaning of touch to the individual is not clear cut. Neither pain nor touch can be measured in precisely the same way as temperature and drug dosage, though analogue scales may be very useful both in research and practice (Bondestam et al. 1987). Only each individual patient can say what constitutes for him or her tolerable and intolerable levels of pain or whether therapy, of whatever kind, has reduced the awareness of pain. As the above study demonstrated nurses tend to underestimate the degree of pain experienced by patients and to overestimate the therapeutic effect of drugs. When we get to notions of 'unruffling the field' and 'modulation of energy' (Wright 1987) we would, perhaps, do well to submit such hypotheses to the most rigorous scientific testing. They are expressed in what appears to be a scientific format rather than in terms of patients' experiences, beliefs and understandings and must, therefore, expect to be investigated through experimental research.

There have been a lot of attempts to study the environment, particularly in so far as it touches psychiatric patients, where the concern has been not simply with the physical environment but with the social milieu. The therapeutic community as an exercise in the deliberate management of patients though group living goes back at least to the late 1940s. Moos (1973) has categorised environments within the framework of human ecology in a wide-ranging typology which goes far beyond what nurses normally think of when they concern themselves with the patients' immediate ward environment.

Comfort is one of the less studied aspects of therapeutic nursing. There is, for example, work on comfort and pain (Eland 1988), the comfort needs of cancer patients (Fleming et al. 1987) and on self care and comfort (Richeson and Huch 1988). Cameron (1988) explored the concept with patients while they were still in hospital using informal interviews and observation. In her abstract she writes, 'Current thought appeared to relegate comfort to an inferior position of soothing rather than to a dynamic process that altered the uncomfortable state'. She uses a grounded theory approach and develops the concept of integrative balancing to describe the process by which patients attempt to redress the disequilibrium which they experience in hospital. While one might question her assertion that 'It could reasonably be said that the motive underlying almost every patient action was a striving to increase comfort', her work does suggest that comfort is a high priority for patients and that nurses may fail to recognise that patients are actively in pursuit of comfort and can be helped or hindered by the extent to which nurses share their understanding of what is involved.

Some things can be shown to 'work' without our being able to explain why in our present state of knowledge or understanding. That may be an adequate basis for adoption into practice on a temporary basis, a working hypothesis, but even if only non-invasive activities are involved questions about whether, how and why they work must continue to be asked. Some things do not even need to be proved through nursing research. Nursing research does not, for example, need to prove that institutionalisation may give rise to sensory deprivation (Heron et al. 1954). Nursing research should concentrate, instead, on the application to nursing of such findings generated in other arenas.

OUTCOMES FOR PATIENTS

Advanced nursing practice, therefore, is concerned with the very basics of nursing: with independent practice initiated by nurses related to the core of nursing, with emotional labour, focuses on healing, has a deliberate therapeutic intent and relies on the nurse's use of self. Krulik quoted by Bircumshaw (1988) has stated that 'it is very questionable if the true core of nursing . . . the caring, the interpersonal interaction, ethical judgement, priority decision making etc. can be quantified'. The essential inability to quantify does not mean that these ideas cannot be explored through research. Not long ago doctors would have argued that diagnosis was a matter of specialised knowledge, experience and gut feeling which could not yield to research. The process whereby decisions are made can be extrapolated and used to fuel a computer-based 'expert system'. The resultant diagnostic decisions, which can take into account more information than a doctor can readily manipulate unaided, are more accurate than those based on more traditional methods. Unnecessary operative procedures are avoided and hospital costs reduced (de Dombal 1969). There is no inherent reason why some of the secrets of nursing should not be yielded up in similar ways and using similar methodologies. Nightingale (1859) herself was convinced that these things could be elucidated. 'Let people who have to observe sickness and death look back and try to register in their observation the appearances which have preceded relapse, attack, or death, and not assert that there were none, or that they were not the *right* ones.' Research does not eliminate clinical judgement. It does offer ways in which such judgement may be supported and improved.

While therapeutic nursing may have as its rationale the bringing about of beneficial outcomes for patients the nature of such outcomes and the demonstration that they are beneficial poses problems for both practitioner and researcher. Who is the arbiter of benefit? What is the trade off between short-term and long-term benefit? What happens when nurses and patients disagree about the value of the outcome? Only the patient knows what really works in matters of pain and comfort. But the nurse must also be aware of the objectively dangerous consequences of any attempt to avoid all pain and discomfort.

Many of the subjective outcomes for patients, though they have a value in their own right, probably depend in part for their efficacy on a treatment equivalent of the Hawthorne effect. When nurses spend more time talking to patients (Tarasuk et al. 1965, MacBride 1967) patients' perception of well-being is increased. Many of the reports of good outcomes for alternative physical therapies may simply reflect that they all require time spent together by patient and therapist and it is the longer encounter and the occasion for communication which this affords which is the important element.

At the individual level, the process of nursing is assessing the problem, deciding on appropriate nursing intervention and evaluating the outcome. Where the same time of intervention can be shown to have similar outcomes for other patients we have moved into researching the practice. Case comparison is a perfectly legitimate way of developing knowledge. In principle, nursing process documentation should offer a rich harvest for clinical nursing research. In practice, the information recorded is often not detailed or accurate enough to provide data for research. Computerised storage and retrieval systems at ward level could bring about a major change in the quality of available data. Information on outcomes and evaluation of the contribution of the nursing intervention to that outcome is rarely made explicit (Report of the Nursing Process Evaluation Working Group 1986). If practitioners are unable to specify the effects of what they do then it is unlikely that research into nursing outcomes for patients will get very far. Not only is there a need for greater clarity in determining what is independent nursing intervention, but there is also a need for work to be done in specifying outcomes which might be directly attributed to nurses and their work.

There are outcomes of varying order. There are long-term objective outcomes, such as five-year survival rates of QUALYS (Quality of Life Years), in which the impact of nursing is assumed to be negligible, and short-term subjective outcomes, such as a terminally ill patient feeling comfortable and pain-free for several hours, in which it is allowed that nursing may have made a major contribution. The former may find their way into performance indicators while the latter is likely to remain at the level of an entry in the nursing record. It is, none the less, an important outcome of nursing care for that patient.

The problem for nursing is how to present such small-scale outcomes in order that the value of nursing be recognised beyond the immediate situation.

In addition, many people other than the nurse are involved in the care of patients. They, too, feel that they have a unique therapeutic relationship with patients. It is not easy to see what part of the overall outcome for patients might be attributed to the input of nurses. Objective outcome measures, such as length of stay, re-admission rates, survival rates, may be a useful way of approaching the overall effectiveness of a hospital, ward, service or a specific therapeutic regimen, whether the latter is initiated by doctor or nurse, but have little to contribute to the understanding of the process. Nursing is a process. It is the way in which care is given which is the *independent* variable. But we have to demonstrate that the caring is in the quality and that the quality of the caring matters.

IMPLEMENTING RESEARCH FINDINGS IN PRACTICE

It is received wisdom that the findings from nursing research do not inform practice. Brett (1988) has looked at the diffusion of research-based practices among qualified nurses in the USA and has shown that most nurses are aware of some items of validated practice, such as closed sterile drainage systems, but that relatively few know about others, such as the idea of deliberative nursing, an approach of skilled communication which allows the nurse effectively to ascertain the patient's real needs. There is, moreover, a gap between knowing about a practice and actually using it all the time. Though 94% of her respondents knew about the importance of regular changing of the intravenous site only 27% claimed always to ensure regular change was carried out in practice. Although 34% knew about deliberative nursing only 9% claimed always to make use of the technique in assessing patients.

It could be claimed that looking at items of practice in this way merely confirms the shopping-list approach to both practice and research and that we should be looking at different ways of exploring how far research does inform work in real practice settings. The focus should not be on the individual nurse but on behaviour in the place of work.

Various explanations have been put forward for the research-practice gap. Nurses do not make use of research for a variety of reasons enumerated by Hunt (1981). Perhaps one of the additional reasons is that they do not subscribe to the view of 'nurse as scientist': a concept which Kennedy (1980) maintains has led medicine to take the wrong path. Moira Hunt (1987) sees the problem in terms of nurses' lack of ownership of information and involvement in the research process. Action research is often put forward as *the* method for nursing as it involved practitioners but does not always appear to yield results commensurate with the effort involved.

It is not that the positivist approach is never appropriate for nursing research but that not all problems to which practitioners seek solutions can be addressed in this way. Susman and Evered (1978) argue that 'positivist science is deficient for generating knowledge for use in solving problems that members of organisations face'. Importantly for our concern with why research findings are not implemented in practice is their contention that it is because positivist science leads to research being seen as an 'accumulation of social facts that can be drawn on by practitioners when they are ready to apply them. This conception encourages a separation of theory from practice because published research is read more by producers of research than by practitioners'.

If we are worried about the need to take on a holistic view of the patient we need also to concern ourselves with a holistic notion of nursing in which not only is research and practice not separated but also researcher and practitioner are not always different people. The creation of nursing development units and the growth in opportunities for practitioners to undertake research training courses tailored to their specific needs indicate that the inherent dangers of such a split are being recognised and action taken to bridge the chasm before it gets too wide.

Neither the term therapeutic nursing nor deliberative nursing figure as yet in the expression of priorities for research. As our perceptions of what constitutes nursing and our understanding of the nature of the nurse-patient relationship change, so must our notions of what constitutes appropriate and worthwhile research. Not only shall we ask different 'research questions' but we shall also draw from different theoretical perspectives. It is the nature of the question posed, not the problem identified, that determines the appropriateness of theory, methodology, research design, tools and tests.

Jonathan Miller (1989), in speaking of film editors, said 'As with any hands-on craft the editor would not be able to spell out the principles on which he works'. It is one of the tasks of nursing research to distil such principles from observation of the craft-in-practice, to articulate them in clear and unambiguous terms and to validate them against the experiential knowledge of the nurse and the patient.

ACKNOWLEDGEMENTS

I am grateful to Philip Burnard, Sandy Kirkman and Paul Wainwright for their constructive criticism on the draft and to several other colleagues for tracking down elusive references.

REFERENCES

Binnie, A. (1987) 'Primary nursing: structural changes' *Nursing Times*, **83**(39), 36–7.

Bircumshaw, D. (1989) 'How can we compare graduate and non-graduate nurses? A review of the literature', *Journal of Advanced Nursing*, **14** 438–43.

Bond, J. and Bond, S. (1982) *Clinical Nursing Research Priorities: A Delphi Survey*, Health Care Research Unit, University of Newcastle upon Tyne and Northern Regional Health Authority.

Bondestam, E., Hovgren, K., Johansson, F.G., Jern, S., Herlitz, J. and Holmberg, S. (1987) 'Pain assessment by patients and nurses in the early stages of acute myocardial infarction', *Journal of Advanced Nursing*, **12** 677–82.

Brett, J.L. (1987) 'Use of nursing practice research findings', Nursing Research **36**(6), 344–9.

Cameron, B.L., (1988) *The Nature of Comfort to Hospitalized Patients*, unpublished MSc thesis, University of Wales.

Department of Health and Social Security (1989) *DHSS Handbook of Research and Development 1988*, HMSO, London.

Dombal, F.T. de (1979) 'Computers and the Surgeon', *Surgery Annual*, **11** 33–57.

Eland, J.M. (1988) 'Pain management and comfort', *Journal of Gerontological Nursing*, **14**(4), 10–15.

Ersser, S. (1988) 'Nursing beds and nursing therapy' in Pearson, A. (ed.) *Primary Nursing*, Croom Helm, Beckenham.

Fleming, C. *et al.* (1987) 'A study of the comfort needs of patients with advanced cancer', *Cancer Nursing*, **10**(5) 237–43.

Harlow, H.F. and Harlow, M.K. (1966) 'Learning to love', *American Scientist*, **54** 244–72.

Heron, W., Doane, B.K. and Scott, T.H. (1956) 'Visual disturbances after prolonged perceptual isolation', *Canadian Journal of Psychology* **10** 13–16.

Hochschild, A.R. (1983) *The Managed Heart: Commercialisation of Human Feeling*, University of California Press, Berkeley.

Hockey, L., (1989) 'Therapeutic nursing: its development and its debut', paper read at the First National Conference on Therapeutic Nursing held in Oxford on March 22nd 1989.

Hockey, L. (1989) 'The birth and development of two research units: similarities and contrasts', paper read at the RCN Conference on Research in Nursing: Retrospect and Prospect held in London on September 12th 1989.

Hunt, J. (1981) 'Indicators for nursing practice: the use of research findings', *Journal of Advanced Nursing*, **6** 189–94.

Hunt, M. (1987) 'The process of translating research findings into practice', *Journal of Advanced Nursing*, **12** 101–10.

Institute of Medical Ethics (1989) *Bulletin*, (49) p. 6.

Jennings, B.M. and Rogers, S. (1988) 'Merging nursing research and practice: a case of multiple identities', *Journal of Advanced Nursing*, **13** 752–8.

Keller, E. and Bzdek, V.M. (1986) 'Effects of therapeutic touch on tension headache pain', *Nursing Research*, **35**(2) 101–5.

Kennedy, I. (1980) 'The Reith Lectures: unmasking medicine, *The Listener*.

Lathlean, J. and Farnish, S. (1984) *The Ward Sister Training Project*, Nursing Education Research Unit, King's College, London.

Lucker, K.A. (1983) 'An evaluation of health visitors' visits to elderly women' in Wilson-Barnett, J.L. (ed.) *Nursing Research: Ten Studies in Patient Care*, John Wiley & Sons Ltd., Chichester.

McBride, M.A.B. (1967) 'Nursing approach, pain and relief: an exploratory experiment', *Nursing Research*, **11** 337–41.

McMahon, R. (1989) Therapeutic nursing, theory and practice, paper read at the First National Conference on Therapeutic Nursing held in Oxford on March 22nd 1989.

Menzies, I. (1960) 'A case-study in the functioning of social systems as a defence against anxiety', *Human Relations*, **13**(2) 95–123.

Miller, J. (1989) *Equinox* (Channel 4 TV programme).

Moos, R. 'Conceptualisation of human environments', *American Psychologist*, **28** 652–65.

Muetzel, P.-A. (1988) 'Therapeutic nursing' in Pearson, A. (ed.), *Primary Nursing*, Croom Helm, London.

Netten, A. (1988) *The effect of the design of residential homes in creating dependency among confused elderly residents*, DP 562, University of Kent, Canterbury.

Nightingale, F. (1859) *Notes on Nursing*, (republished 1980), Churchill Livingstone, Edinburgh.

Nuffield Provincial Hospitals Trust (1954) *The Work of Nurses in Hospital Wards*, (The Goddard Report), NPHT, London.

Pearson, A. (1988) 'Primary nursing', in Pearson, A. (ed.) *Primary Nursing*, Croom Helm, London.

Report of the Committee on Nursing (1972) HMSO, London.

Report of the Nursing Process Evaluation Working Group to the DHSS Research Liaison Group (1986) ed. Haywood, J., Nurse Education Research Unit, Report No. 5, King's College, London.

Report of the Royal Commission on the National Health Service, (1979) HMSO, London.

Revans, R.W. (1964) 'The morale and effectiveness of general hospitals', in McLachlan, G. (ed.) *Problems and Progress in Medical Care*, Oxford University Press, Oxford.

Richeson, M. and Huch, M. (1988) 'Self-care and comfort: a framework for nursing practice', *New Zealand Nursing Journal*, **81**(6) 26–7.

Robinson, J., Stilwell, J., Hawley, C. and Hempstead, N. (1989) *The Role of the Support Worker in the Ward Health Care Team*, Nursing Policy Studies 6, Nursing Policies Studies Centre and Health Services Research Unit, University of Warwick.

Smith, P., (1988) 'The emotional labour of nursing', *Nursing Times*, **84**(44) 50–1.

Smith, P. (1989) 'Emotional labour, nursing work and the research process: measuring quality of life', paper given at the Royal College of Nursing Research Society Annual Conference, University College, Swansea, April 14th–16th, 1989.

Susman, G.I. and Evered, R.D. (1978) 'An assessment of the scientific merits of action research', *Administrative Science Quarterly*, **23** 582–603.

Tarasuk, M.B., Rhymes, J.P. and Leonard, R.C. (1965) 'An experimental test of the importance of communication skills for effective nursing', in Skipper, J.K. and Leonard, R.C. (eds) *Social Interaction and Patient Care*, Lippincott, Philadelphia.

West Birmingham Community Health Council (1989) *Ethical Committees*, Birmingham.

Wharton, A. and Pearson, A. (1988) 'Nursing and intimate physical care – the key to therapeutic nursing', in Pearson, A. (ed.) *Primary Nursing*, Croom Helm, Beckenham.

Wright, S.M. (1987) 'The use of therapeutic touch in the management of pain', *Nursing Clinics of North America*, **22**(3) 705–14.

Zorza, V. and Zorza, R. (1980) *A Way to Die*, André Deutsch, London.

Chapter 7

An exploration of touch and its use in nursing

ELIZABETH TUTTON

INTRODUCTION

Touch and its importance to the development of human beings and their continued well-being has been well documented (Montague 1971, Barnett 1972). The act of touching, according to Watson (1975), is an 'intentional physical contact between two or more individuals'. This definition is limited as it merely describes touch as an outward physical action. In this chapter the definition of touch is expanded to include the transference of feelings and energy between two or more individuals.

There are many obvious examples of nurses using touch in their work. Nurses hold hands with patients who are experiencing a traumatic procedure, such as having their stitches or a drain removed. They touch patients in order to lift them into more comfortable positions. Touch is also necessary when nurses facilitate the relearning of dressing or walking skills by patients. The nature of nursing work allows nurses the privilege of close bodily contact at the very beginning of a relationship with a patient. Touch often occurs at the first meeting. Other examples are a light touch on the arm to reassure a patient, or in the performance of admission procedures such as taking a pulse or blood pressure. Often the first contact is of a more intimate nature and involves the provision of help with toileting or cleaning the patient's body. Touch is therefore an integral part of nursing care, but how frequently do we as nurses consider its use? Do we always use touch appropriately? Are we using touch to its fullest potential in order to provide high quality nursing care? Le

May and Redfern (1987) demonstrate that in one elderly care setting the majority of touch provided by nurses was related to the performance of a procedure. This suggests that other forms of touch may be under-utilised.

The use of touch in nursing is not a new topic for discussion. Estabrooks (1987) provides evidence of a well developed use of touch in American and Canadian nursing literature in the early 19th century. Currently there is a resurgence of interest in touch and its use in nursing as evidenced in recent British literature (Harrison 1986, Sims 1986b, Le May 1986, Turton 1989). There may be several reasons for this interest. The first may be concerned with an attempt to counteract the dehumanising effects of a patient's stay in a modern hospital. Murphy (1984) indicates the highly stressful nature of a 'high tech' hospital environment which can adversely affect patients' well-being. Naisbett (1982) suggests that nurses are in an ideal position to use touch to provide a high level of personal contact in an alien hospital environment. Secondly nurses are constantly reviewing the principles from which they practise. The current trend in nursing is moving away from a concept of nursing based on a medical model of practice towards practice that encompasses holistic principles (Pearson and Vaughan 1986). The principles of holistic practice, treating the person as a unified whole, underlie most forms of complementary therapy. Similarities between the goals of nursing and those of complementary therapies have led many nurses to use some of these therapies to enhance their nursing practice (Holmes 1986, Tutton 1987, Wise 1989). For example, the use of massage as a form of touch within nursing is increasing. Its use along with other advances in nursing care has been shown significantly to increase the quality of care nurses provide (Pearson et al. 1988).

This chapter is divided into two main parts: the first explores the use of instrumental, expressive and therapeutic touch and the second looks at massage. A general discussion of each form of touch is followed by a brief research critique of some of the major studies investigating these areas. At the same time it is hoped that individuals will explore their own beliefs and values about touch and how they use it in their own practice. A series of exercises is provided throughout for this purpose. The reader is also given the opportunity to experience massage in the form of an example of a foot massage. Finally, methods of evaluating the use of touch in practice are considered.

INSTRUMENTAL, EXPRESSIVE AND THERAPEUTIC TOUCH

Exercise 1.   Write down a brief description of three different incidents where you have touched a patient. What were you hoping to achieve by touching them?

The most recent nursing research places touch within a framework of communication theory, viewing touch as a form of non verbal communication (Sims 1986a, Tutton 1987, Le May and Redfern 1987). Estabrooks (1987) questions this deductive approach. From a review of early nurses' writings she suggests that touch should be viewed as an integral part of the concept of comfort. The provision of comfort in the form of touch was a key role of the nurse that appears to have been neglected in more recent literature.

The use of touch in nursing according to Sims (1986a) can be divided into four categories:

1. Instrumental touch;
2. Expressive touch;
3. Therapeutic touch;
4. Systematic touch.

Watson (1975) defines instrumental touch as a deliberate physical contact made as part of a procedure, such as performing an aseptic technique, or supporting a patient learning to walk again. Expressive touch is seen as spontaneous and affective in nature. A hug to comfort a patient who is feeling unhappy is demonstrating expressive touch. Therapeutic touch involves the transference of energy from one person to another with the intention to heal (Krieger 1978). Systematic touch could be seen as synonymous with massage, which can be defined as a purposeful manipulation of the soft tissues of the body with the intention of enhancing the receiver's well-being.

Exercise 2. Can you identify these forms of touch in your three descriptions?

Instrumental touch

Instrumental touch is essential for the performance of nursing tasks. Watson (1975) assumed that touch in health professionals is primarily instrumental in nature. Le May and Redfern (1987) observed 1420 touches during 318 interactions between nurse and patient. Of these 1216 (85.63%) were instrumental and 181 (12.75%) were expressive and 23 (1.62%) indefinable. This study had a sample of 30 patients and took place on a long stay elderly care ward. Although generalisations beyond this care setting cannot be made this study provides weighty evidence to support Watson's assumption.

The emphasis on the use of instrumental touch may relate to the nurses' working patterns. A system of task allocation, where nurses are given one or more tasks to perform to a large group of patients, may mean that no one person is aware of the interrelated nature of the patient's needs. The scope for appreciation of instances where other forms of touch may improve a patient's well-being could be limited. Melia (1987) suggests that student nurses are quickly socialised into the ward culture with its emphasis on getting the work finished. This ethos may also reduce the opportunities for forms of touch other than instrumental. Other factors such as the layout of the ward, ward furniture, patients' diagnosis, cultural background and personality of the nurse and patient may also conspire to limit touch to its instrumental form.

Exercise 3. Identify factors in your work patterns and work environment that might make you use only instrumental touch.

Expressive touch

Locsin (1984) considers that touch affects people's feelings of value and worth, their integration and ego integrity. Johnson (1985) sees touch as a behaviour that communicates comfort, love, security and warmth with implications for physical survival as well as emotional self esteem. Barnett (1972a) indicates that people convey their inner feelings and reactions through touch to others. Locsin (1984) and Goodykoontz (1979) describe touch as a sense through which one person shares themselves with another. Goodykoontz continues that touch can communicate caring, well-being and facilitate recovery and acceptance of a diagnosis. Seaman (1982) also sees touch as beneficial as it carries messages of acceptance and caring. Touching in a caring manner is seen as therapeutic by Ernst and Shaw (1980). It also has the potential to communicate trust according to Hollinger (1980). Click (1986) has demonstrated that expressive touch has the potential to decrease, though not significantly, anxiety in patients who have had a myocardial infarction.

Touch can also be used to convey negative emotions or to communicate distance and non-involvement. Avoidance of touch may be interpreted by the patient as the nurse's dislike of that patient (Goodykoontz 1979). Other patients may feel uncomfortable when touched (Seaman 1982, Goodykoontz 1979).

Exercise 4. How do you feel when you touch other people? Write down your thoughts.

Ask someone to touch you. Discuss what you felt with them. Did what they intended you to feel match up with what you felt?

Practise using different ways of touching and explore the effects of your touch in relation to what you intended the person to feel.

Therapeutic touch

Therapeutic touch, or the laying on of hands, is an ancient form of healing. It involves the transference of 'energy' known as Chi in China and Prana in India, from the healer to the sick person. Its use in nursing was pioneered by Dolores Krieger in the 1970s. Krieger was impressed by the work of Grad and Smith, who used controlled experiments to assess the effect of Colonel Estabany, a well-known healer, on the healing of skin wounds in mice (Krieger 1975). Grad et al. (1961) found mice treated by Colonel Estabany healed significantly faster. The same team found a comparable effect when barley seeds were treated in the same manner: the height of the seedlings and yield of plant material was significantly higher. Krieger (1975) reports on her studies using haemoglobin as the dependent variable. In all her three studies haemoglobin values were significantly higher after treatment with therapeutic touch. Krieger then went on to test her assumption that anyone with a fairly healthy body and a strong intention to help or heal ill people could become healers. The same research study was then carried out using 32 registered nurses who had been taught healing. The results confirmed that ordinary nurses taught therapeutic touch can significantly affect haemoglobin levels in ill people. Husband (1988) argues strongly for the use of therapeutic touch and its incorporation into nursing practice. She proposes that therapeutic touch with its ability to produce a relaxation response and pain relief has many possible applications in patient care. Turton (1988) said that therapeutic touch is an 'eminently suitable therapy for nurses to incorporate into their care'.

Exercise 5.   Find yourself a quiet place and make yourself comfortable. Close your eyes. Place both your hands together as in the traditional sign of prayer. Now move your hands until they are 2 cm apart. Concentrate your mind on the space between your hands. Then slowly move your hands until they are 4 cm apart and then bring them together until they are nearly touching. Repeat this action for about three minutes.

What did you feel? Ask your friends to try this exercise and share your experiences. (For more information about this exercise read Krieger (1979), Chapter 3.)

A review of the research studies on touch

A large study looking at where and which patients, health professionals touch, was undertaken by Barnett (1972b). Using observation over a four-week period on randomly selected wards and rooms, all unnecessary touch that took place was recorded. Information gathered showed that registered nurses touched patients the most with the female members giving 85% more touch then the male members. The age of the patient was related to the amount of touch, with decreasing touch with increasing age. Most touch was given to 26- to 33-year-olds, and 72% of touches occurred on patients who were 18 to 33 years old. The six to 17-year-olds and 42- to 49-year-olds were not touched at all. Touch levels were higher in paediatrics, labour rooms and intensive care. Barnett considered this to be related to the high stress levels in these areas. The hand was the commonest place of touch, receiving 60%. The amount of touch a patient received was also based on their condition with 70% of those touched being considered to be good or fair. This study gives us very useful descriptive data, but lacks any evidence of inter-observer reliability testing.

Further studies have been undertaken with pre-experimental and quasi-experimental designs, using different subject samples. Lorensen (1983) undertook a small qualitative study using post testing only, on 12 primagravida women during labour. The sample was one of convenience, with no randomisation and there was little control over the amount of touch the control women received. The investigator administered a high degree of touch during labour to the experimental group. The control group received instrumental touch only. An author-designed questionnaire of which there was no evidence of reliability or validity, was administered between 24 and 36 hours later. The results showed no significant differences. However in answer to the question who was most helpful, four chose the nurse in the experimental group, one chose the nurse in the control group. Five subjects in the experimental group said that holding their hand was the most important thing the nurse did. Five subjects in the experimental group found massage relieved low back discomfort.

Aguilera (1967), using a quasi-experimental design with 36 psychiatric patients, investigated the use of physical contact and verbal interactions. The experimental group received simple appropriate touch with verbal commands whilst the control group received no touch. A subject attitude questionnaire was given before and after intervention and an observation sheet was filled in. There was no evidence of reliability, validity testing of the tools or inter-observer reliability and not all patient variables were considered. No statistical tests of significance were used on the results. Aguilera claims that there was increased verbal interaction, rapport and approach behaviour particularly after the eighth day in the touch group. There was no evidence of a greater increase in verbal interaction in the evening shift. The degree of comfort of nurses was positively correlated with the degree of comfort of the subjects. There was also a higher rate of acceptance of schizophrenic subjects compared with depressive subjects by nurses. Aguilera also found a significant correlation between age and amount of touch, with younger subjects receiving higher comfort and acceptance ratings from nurses.

Taking Aguilera's study one step further, Langland and Panicucci (1982) designed a study to see if touch, while giving a verbal request, increased attention, verbal response and action response. They used a convenience sample of 32 elderly female patients who had been confused for six months or more. The patients were assessed using known tools and allocated randomly to each group. The experimental group received touch with a verbal request and the control group received just the verbal request, the subjects were assessed for attention using an author-designed tool which showed no evidence of reliability or validity testing. There was also no evidence of investigator and observer reliability using this tool. The subject's verbal response was tape recorded and physical action documented by the investigator and observer. Results from this study showed significantly increased attention and non-verbal response when touch was used. The subjects showed no increase in relevant verbal response and no increase in appropriate action response. Other authors using a case study approach have found touch increases the verbal and action response. Burnside (1973) worked with a group of six elderly regressive patients with chronic brain syndrome. Using touch as part of the therapy, she increased the amount of non-verbal and verbal communication within the group. Preston (1973) also gives a case study of touch used with a request increasing the non-verbal and action response in an elderly gentleman with organic brain syndrome.

There are two studies on touch with critically ill patients. A well designed study by McCorkle (1974) looked at 60 seriously ill patients randomly allocating them to an experimental group, who received touch to the wrist while talking to the investigator. The control group received the verbal interaction but no touch. The questionnaire used had face validity and reliability, the observers had interrater reliability and a tape recording made of the verbal interaction was analysed using Bale's Interaction Process Analysis. There were a number of significant results. A greater number of the patients in the experimental group responded positively with facial expressions. Correspondingly, a greater number of control patients responded negatively with facial expressions. The experimental group had significantly more neutral movements and fewer negative movements. Analysis of the verbal responses showed that significantly more of the experimental group responded positively, in fact, 93.3% of the control group, 70% responded positively. Responses to the question, 'Was the nurse interested in you?' were approximately the same for both groups. Of the experimental group 90% said 'Yes' and 87% of the control group said 'Yes'. ECG readings were also taken but proved inconclusive. The other study performed on critically ill patients was by Knable (1981). This study was based on a qualitative approach using hand holding when it naturally occurs and describing what happens. The author combines this with pre and post physiological measurements. Fifteen subjects and 12 nurses were used, with the investigator as measurer and observer. The nurses chose two periods in four hours when they would normally hold hands with the patient. The results showed that hand holding lasted up to three minutes and was used primarily to provide emotional support and to establish rapport. Of 306 non-verbal interactions, 222 were positive and 85 negative. The vital signs proved to be inconclusive.

To summarise, most of the studies to date have been experimental in design, with convenience samples which have been randomly allocated into experimental and control groups. There has been a lack of reliability and validity testing of tools and inter observer reliability apart from McCorkle (1974). The results indicate that most touches occur to the hand and the amount of touches decreases with age (Barnett 1972). Hand holding enhances positive, non-verbal response in critically ill patients (Knable 1981) and is most important to mothers in labour (Lorensen 1983). A verbal request accompanied by touch can increase verbal and non-verbal responses (Langland and Panicucci 1982, Aguilera 1967 and McCorkle 1974). Finally, physiological measures such as vital signs and ECGs produce inconclusive evidence. Lader and Mathews (1970) question the efficacy of using physiological indices to measure autonomic changes at low levels of arousal. They claim that patient variables, obtrusive devices and artifacts can affect the measurements.

A review of the research studies on therapeutic touch

Three recent studies have looked at the effect of therapeutic touch on anxiety states. Randolph (1984) induced anxiety on his 60 healthy subjects in the form of a silent film. Using a quasi-experimental design the experimental group received therapeutic touch during the film while the control group received physical touch. Pre and post measures of skin conductance level, muscle tension level and peripheral skin temperature were recorded. Both groups showed a physiological stress response to the film but there were no differences between the two groups. It could be that the stimulus was too strong for therapeutic touch to be effective. Normally it takes place in a quiet relaxed environment with minimal external stimulus for healer and healee. There was also no evidence of the practitioner's ability to practise this art.

Another researcher, Heidt (1981), chose a population with known high anxiety scores, a sample of 100 patients on a cardiovascular unit. Three groups were used, one who received therapeutic touch, one casual touch (pulse taking) and one with no touch but with verbal interaction. Heidt recorded pre intervention and post intervention state A anxiety scores using Spielberger's self-evaluation questionnaire. The results indicated that the therapeutic touch group experienced a significant decrease in anxiety and had significantly lower scores than the casual touch and non-touch group. The control interventions can, however, be criticised. The casual touch group could have mimicked therapeutic touch to make a truer control and the non-touch group brought a new factor, verbal communication, into the design which as the author discusses allowed the patients to bring up concerns that could not be dealt with in the time available. This in turn could adversely affect their anxiety scores.

To make a tighter research design, Quinn (1984) used two groups, one receiving non-contact therapeutic touch and the other receiving a mimicked version of therapeutic touch. Quinn trained the assistants and then filmed them and tested to see if a panel of judges could tell which ones were using therapeutic touch and which ones were not. Analysis showed no correlation, hence it was proved impossible visually to tell the difference. Pre and post anxiety states were taken, using Spielberger's self-evaluation questionnaire, of 60 patients on a cardiovascular unit. Possible bias could be introduced to the study from the seven different nurses giving the treatments and there was no control for the different anxiety state levels in each group. However, the results still showed a signficant decrease in post-state anxiety scores in patients treated with non-contact therapeutic touch.

MASSAGE IN NURSING

The literature suggests that touch is a means of communicating or sending messages from person to person. Massage as a form of touch has the same effect. Auckett (1979) sees massage as an expression of love through loving, caring and touching. She feels that massage can promote mother-baby bonding, and sets up a metaphysical energy flow between them. It calms unsettled, irritable and colicky babies, by giving them pleasure, awareness, gentleness, closeness and relaxation. Hefferman et al. (1984) also believe that massage is of high value in establishing the mother-baby relationship. Debelle (1981) uses massage in a clinic for babies that are causing their parents some distress. The babies are considered to be uncuddly, irritable, poor feeders, constant criers or sleep fighters. Debelle uses massage successfully to improve the communication between the parents and babies. She claims that massage helps the parents to be:

1. more aware of the babies' needs;
2. tuned into the babies' feelings and responses;
3. able to reassure the baby by maximum skin contact that the environment is safe;
4. able to help the baby relax;
5. able to relax themselves.

Jackson (1985) considers touch to be therapeutic and suggests that it should be given in a structured manner on a regular basis. She recommends massage and says it allows verbal interaction, improvement and maintenance of emotional well-being, relief of pain and muscle tension, establishment of a unifying bond between nurse and patient and socialisation through one-to-one contact. Hollinger (1980) suggests that nurses can communicate trust through back rubs and reinforce feelings of well-being and self-worth. From his experience of using massage with orthopaedic patients Mason (1988) said that massage provided the opportunity for the patient to discuss his problems with his nurse. The nurse also uses the massage sessions to pick up cues about the patient's physical and mental state. Wharton and Pearson (1988) consider massage to facilitate the development of a close nurse-patient relationship. They provide a case study of a patient who was helped to cope with a painful procedure through the use of massage.

Massage is contra-indicated according to Joachim (1983b) where there are skin lesions, blood clots, fractures or extreme arthritic pain. Breakey (1982) also indicates that patients on bed rest should not have their legs massaged to prevent mobilisation of a thrombosis or emboli formation.

Most authors consider that massage may have a relaxing effect on the subject (Jackson 1977, Joachim 1983a, Breakey 1982). By association, massage may have physiological effects. Joachim (1983a) suggests that massage increases the flexibility of muscles, increases circulation by dilating blood vessels, facilitates the removal of waste products and prevents contractures and tension. Breakey (1982) agrees with Joachim and adds that massage promotes lymphatic drainage, benefits connective tissue and increases fibre networks, presumably by improving venous return. It also decreases oedema and post-operative pooling of blood and improves gastro-intestinal activity. Joachim (1983a) also claims that massage decreases the use of pain and sleeping medication.

Exercise 6. Consider the factors (those that relate to yourself, your patient, or the environment) that might influence your use of massage in your area of practice.

These factors might relate to yourself in terms of your sexuality, the clothes you wear, or maybe how you perceive your role. The patients' diagnoses, their appearance, or how they behave might be influencing factors. Environmental factors might be that there is too much noise, or too much light.

Explore these factors and consider alternatives that might facilitate the use of massage in your area of practice.

A review of the research studies on massage

Research studies that systematically collect data on the physiological and psychological effects of massage are few and far between. Only seven were isolated from a literature search. Each of these studies had different subject sample and covered different outcome measures.

A study by Kaufmann (1964) looked at the physiological and subjective responses of 36 patients who received a back rub. Each subject acted as their own control with half receiving the back rub first and half receiving it second. The control period of rest was undertaken on another day which could lead to bias if the patients' feelings or condition had changed with time. There were also four nurses administering the massage and three nurses taking recordings, which would introduce some variations in technique. The study provided no indication of random assignment of patients to each group. The results were disappointing with no statistical significance between the physiological measurements of each group. However, 31 subjects gave strongly positive responses to their back rubs.

Using ten healthy subjects, Barr and Tazlitz (1970) attempted to discover if physiological relaxation occurred with massage. Each subject undertook six consecutive sessions of alternating massage and a control rest period. The results were inconclusive and certainly gave no indication of a relaxation response. Initially systolic and diastolic pressure decreased during massage, yet at the end of the massage there was an increase in systolic and a small decrease in diastolic pressure. Heart rate increased during massage and body temperature decreased as a result of increased sweating. However there were no discernible trends in skin temperature, pupil diameter or axillary sweating.

Another study using 32 healthy female subjects was undertaken by Longworth (1982). The author used a pseudo-experimental pre and post intervention test design, she did not have a control session and the intervention was a massage session. Pre and post Spielberger state anxiety inventories were taken and pre as well as post measurements of heart rate, blood pressure, galvanic skin response and muscle tension. The results indicated a significant decrease in state anxiety scores and no significant changes in physiological measures.

Joachim (1983b) also considered physiological factors and found that, after massage, pulse rates decreased by five to 20 beats per minute. Blood pressure readings were inconclusive. Joachim's design, however, was a weak, pre-experimental one-group pre-post test design, and so strong inferences cannot be made. The sample was 15 randomly selected patients with inflammatory bowel disease. Each patient had four sessions with 30 minutes of deep breathing exercises and 45 minutes of body massage. Pre and post interviews were conducted on four aspects of well-being. The design of the study made it impossible to isolate the effect of deep breathing from that of massage. However, useful qualitative data was obtained using techniques that could be incorporated into care planning. Nine patients demonstrated an increased ability to sleep, and nine patients also felt more in control of their pain. Fourteen patients said they were more aware of the difference between feeling stressed and feeling relaxed. Thirteen patients were better able to calm themselves and 14 patients said massage helped them feel more relaxed.

A more recent but severely limited study by Rowlands (1984) had a sample of 24 elderly patients. The design was pre-experimental post test only, with questionnaires given to all the staff and subjects in the home at the end of the study. The subjects were put into three groups: one had therapeutic touch twice a day, one group had it once a day, and the third group had nothing. Therapeutic touch was not adequately defined but turned out to be massage. The subjects were not randomly allocated and because of the three group design, there were only small numbers in each group. The nurses giving the intervention were the nurses on duty at the time so over the six-week period the intervention was not standardised. There was no reliability or validity testing of the questionnaire and all the staff knew exactly who had the intervention and how often. The results were very positive but must be considered in light of the design. The mood of the experimental subjects was lightened in the first four weeks and they had greater positive behavioural responses. Both experimental groups showed an increase in sociability towards the domestics in weeks two to six. Of the nurses 78.3% believed the massage benefited the residents in the study, while 64% of the residents said they had a reduction in muscle tension and 65% had assisted movement. Finally, 95% of the residents felt that massage was of value to them.

In a study on the effect of teaching mothers to massage their babies to establish if it improved infant development, Booth et al. (1985) assigned primiparas and their infants to three groups: a powder massage group, a non-powder massage group and a control group. Each child had pre and post testing using Bayley scales of infant development, nursing child assessment project teaching scales (NCAP) and post testing of a 30 minute videotape of mother-infant free play and massage session. There was no evidence of random assignment or of observer reliability testing using the aforementioned scales. The results however were statistically inconclusive, but there was considerable positive feedback from all the mothers in the massage group.

The last of the seven studies is a thought-provoking pilot study by Sims (1986a). The sample comprised six female patients with breast cancer undergoing radiotherapy. Each of these patients received three sessions of slow stroke back massage on three consecutive days, followed by three sessions of a control rest period on three consecutive days in the following week. The subjects were randomly allocated into two groups, group one received massage followed by the control periods and group two vice versa. Pre and post measurements of symptom distress (McCorkle 1981) and an author-adapted mood adjective checklist from McNair and Lorr (1964) were taken. The results must be considered in the light of the small sample size but it is interesting that from six patients, 28 spontaneous positive comments were made. Four of the six patients also started spontaneously to talk about their personal concerns. Subjects in group one reported a significant percentage improvement in symptom distress following the massage intervention. However group two showed no difference in percentage improvement following the massage and control interventions. Following the control intervention the percentage improvement in symptom distress for group two was significantly greater than the percentage improvement for group one. For the whole sample a 25% improvement in total symptom distress scores following massage was reported compared with 7.7% improvement following the control intervention. Using the mood checklist group one reported greater improvement on one variable, tense. Whereas group two reported greater improvement in four variables, tranquil, tense, vitality and tired following the massage compared with the control intervention. The whole sample reported an overall mood improvement of 17.9% following the massage compared with 13.3% following the control intervention.

Overall the studies indicate that physiological measurements of massage-induced relaxation are inconclusive. Is this of great importance when adults' subjective responses to well-being after massage are positive in nature? What appears to be needed are some valid and reliable tools to measure well-being followed by large sample studies to establish the effect massage has on well-being.

Principles of giving massage

Massage can be described as the manipulation of soft body tissue by the hand for therapeutic purposes. Different authors suggest variations on the method of massage. Jackson (1977) suggests using four different strokes.

Effleurage or superficial stroking: A longitudinal stroke, light to moderate in pressure which warms the tissues and calms the receiver. It is usually used on the full length of the back and a massage should start and finish with this stroke.

Petrissage or circular or deep transverse stroking: This is a moderate to deep stroke used to feel the muscles and other tissues to discover where tension lies.

Kneading: This is manipulation of underlying tissue using the thumb and fingers of the hand. It is a deep manipulation and may be used on problem areas throughout the massage.

Friction: This is a deep circular motion using the thumb, knuckles or ends of the fingers. The pressure is concentrated in a small area.

The speed at which a massage is performed is of great importance. A rushed massage will cause tension to build up in the receiver. The action should be slow and deliberate and carried out in a relaxed manner so that rapport is established with the subject. It is essential to establish a good rhythm of movement and breathing and that it remains constant throughout the massage. Joachim (1983b) and Jackson (1977) agree on how a massage should be performed. They both indicate that a quiet warm room should be chosen, away from interruptions. Both the giver and receiver need to be in comfortable positions. The masseuse's hands must be washed in warm water, and the oil or medium applied directly on to the hands so that it is warm before being applied to the receiver. Jackson (1977) believes that a holistic massage energy is passed from giver to receiver. The giver should therefore be centred or focused and feel free from all negative feelings, otherwise these will be picked up by the receiver. The receiver also needs to concentrate all her energy on what she is feeling, and in doing so, directs positive feelings and energy towards herself as well as the receiver.

Exercise 7. Centering. Find yourself a quiet place and make yourself comfortable. Close your eyes. Concentrate your mind on your breathing and take slow full deep breaths. Empty your mind of all the worrying tensions of the day and replace them with thoughts of love, peace and happiness. Practise this for a few minutes, several times. For further information about centering read Krieger (1979), Chapter 4.

In practice I have found centering a useful exercise to perform for a few seconds between caring for different patients. It provides a break after the last patient and enables me to concentrate more fully on the following patient.

The massage can last as long as both parties enjoy the exercise. However, Jackson (1977) suggests that 30 minutes is necessary for a full back massage. Breakey (1982) sees a ten minute massage as providing the relaxation necessary to induce a full night's sleep. To massage one part of the body effectively Joachim (1983b) feels ten minutes is also adequate.

Exercise 8. Foot Massage Find yourself a partner with whom

you feel safe and comfortable and who is prepared to join in this exercise. Decide who is going to perform the massage first. It is important that you both experience giving and receiving massage as it is necessary to understand the feelings involved in both giving and receiving touch.

Find a warm comfortable place where you are free from interruptions. You will need some oil. Grape seed oil or almond oil are useful as they are quite light and odourless. Also a towel for resting the feet upon and for wiping excess oil off your hands.

When you are ready, get into positions where you are both comfortable and the feet are accessible. The person who is giving the massage now 'centres' herself using exercise 7. Now place some oil onto your hands and rub them together to warm the oil. Firmly use your hands to smooth oil over the whole of one foot.

For the purpose of this exercise I have planned a set of massage sequences for you to follow, mainly using petrissage. Experienced masseuses do not always follow a set procedure but use their experience and intuition. However by describing a procedure I hope to provide a basis for future massage experiences. Throughout this first massage collect information from the receiver about the effect your touch is having on them. Your partner may want you to press harder or more softly and she may like some areas massaged more than others. In consequent massages the receiver may want to remain quiet and concentrate on enjoying the experience of being massaged. If you should find an area that causes pain, work around the edge of this area. All the time the giver needs to be aware of their breathing and the speed of their strokes.

At the end of the massage repeat the procedure on the other foot, then change roles so that the giver is the receiver and vice versa. Share your experiences with each other. In my experience foot massage has been particularly useful with elderly patients who have experienced strokes or fractured neck of femurs. At the end of a heavy day, much of it spent regaining the skills of walking, they said that foot massage makes them feel relaxed, happy and cared for. I enjoyed giving the massage and felt it increased the level of rapport, and facilitated disclosure between myself and my patients. Once you feel confident performing a foot massage, try massaging one of your patients.

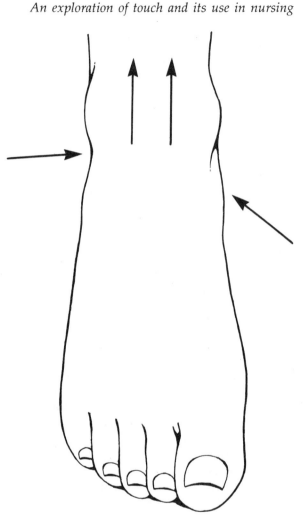

Figure 7.1 Using alternating thumbs stroke the area between the ankle bone in a forwards direction whilst maintaining pressure underneath the ankle bone with your fingers.

Evaluating the massage

Evaluating the effect on the patient is an important part of the massage. The information gained from the evaluation may be used as a basis for making decisions relating to: the massage technique, the timing, duration or frequency of the massage,

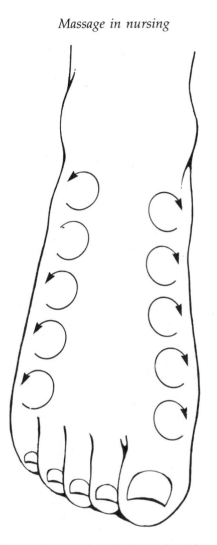

Figure 7.2 Work with your thumbs down the side of the foot using moderate pressure and a circular movement.

or its discontinuation. The two main methods of evaluating massage are to observe the effect it is having on the patient or to ask the patient to provide a verbal report.

Physical observations of vital signs in patients who have received a massage have been shown to be unreliable (Kaufmann 1964, Barr and Tazlitz 1970). Other observable signs

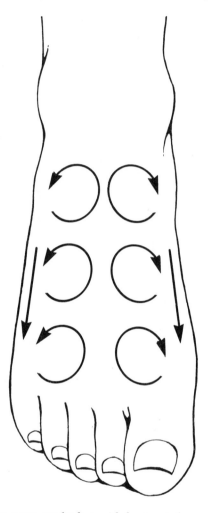

Figure 7.3 Using the same stroke but with larger circles work up the foot with both thumbs and then down the sides.

might be used such as changes in the patients: for example, appearance, depth and speed of breathing, muscle tone, posture, vocal tone, level of activity. Massage will affect people in different ways. Some of my patients fell asleep and others wanted to talk. Whatever observations are made it is useful to have a description of the patient before and after the massage.

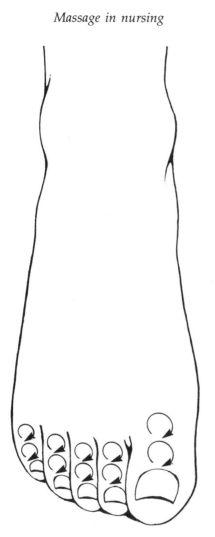

Figure 7.4 Rest one hand underneath the foot whilst the other works on the toes.
Using one hand continue using the circular action up the full length of the toe.
At the end of the toe hold firmly for a few seconds.
Repeat on all five toes.

Asking a patient how he or she feels is a useful way of obtaining information. Tutton (1987) asked elderly patients how they felt after a back massage. They gave responses such

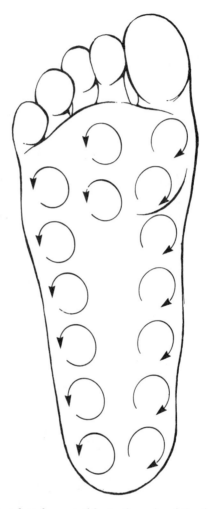

Figure 7.5 Move hands smoothly to the sole of the foot. Work from the heel to the toes using the same circular movements.
To finish place the back of one hand against the sole of the foot and rest for one minute.

as 'that feels comforting, soothing, beautiful, you have a lovely touch', 'I feel relaxed, could fall asleep', 'It's not aching so much, you have eased my backache'. Alternatively if you are using massage to relieve a specific symptom a simple scale may be used to assess the intensity of the symptom before and after the massage. For example, if a patient complains of an awful nagging ache in her left leg, a five-point scale could then be formulated using the patient's own words.

Awful nagging ache	very bad ache	a moderate ache	a slight ache	no ache

Figure 7.6 An example of a five-point scale used to measure symptom relief.

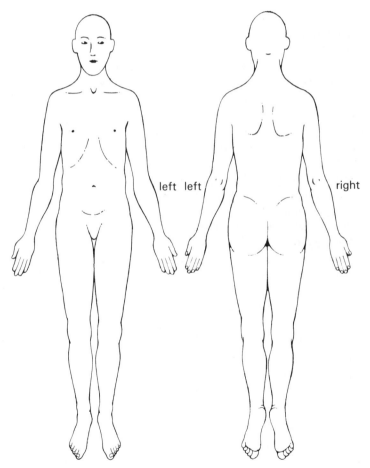

left left   right

Figure 7.7 An example of a body map that can be used to measure the area of discomfort in patients.

Another method used by Tutton (1987) to measure the area of discomfort is the body map. Patients mark on the body map the extent of their discomfort. The area can then be estimated using graph tracing paper and comparisons made.

CONCLUSION

Nurses, as the key providers of intimate physical care and by virtue of their continual presence are in a prime position to use touch to its fullest potential. The selected review of the studies exploring touch have, despite some flaws in the methods, revealed the possible benefits of touch to patients' well-being. Patients appreciate being touched (Kaufmann 1964, Lorensen 1983), touch can increase attention and non-verbal responses (Langland and Panicucci 1982, McCorkle 1974) as well as verbal responses (McCorkle 1974). Therapeutic touch has been shown significantly to reduce anxiety (Heidt 1981, Quinn 1984) as has massage (Longworth 1982). Joachim (1983b) has demonstrated that massage and deep breathing can increase patients' feelings of control as well as their ability to sleep and relax. Patients' symptom distress has also been shown to decrease with massage (Sims 1986a). However there are some interesting findings relating to who nurses touch. For instance the amount of touch patients receive tends to decrease with age, and touch often relates to patients' condition (Aguilera 1967, Barnett 1972). This suggests that the individual's attitude to or beliefs about the patient may affect their use of touch. If touch is to be used to its full potential nurses need to explore their own attitudes and beliefs about their patients and to analyse critic-ally their use of touch in practice. My own positive experiences of using massage with elderly people inspired me to further exploration and I hope other nurses will feel the same.

REFERENCES

Aguilera, D. C. (1967) 'Relationship between physical contact and verbal interaction between nurses and patients', *Journal of Psychiatric Nursing*, 5–21.

Auckett, A. (1979) 'Baby massage an alternative to drugs', *The Australian Nurses' Journal*, **9**(5) 24–7.

Barnett, K. (1972a) 'A theoretical contrast of the concepts of touch as they relate to nursing', *Nursing Research*, **21**(2) 102–9.

Barnett, K. (1972b) 'A survey of the current utilization of touch by health team personnel with hospitalised patients', *International Journal of Nursing Studies*, **9** 195–209.

Barr, J. and Taslitz, N. (1970) 'The influence of back massage on autonomic functions', *Physical Therapy*, **50**(12) 1679–91.

Booth, C. C., Johnston-Crowley, N., Barnard, K. E. (1985) 'Infant massage and exercise, worth the effort?', *American Journal of Maternal and Child Nursing*, **10**(3) 184–9.

Breakey, B. (1982) 'An overlooked therapy you can use ad lib', *R.N.*, 50–4.

Burnside, I. (1973) 'Touching is talking', *Amercian Journal of Nursing*, **73**(12) 2060–3.

Click, M. (1986) 'Caring touch and anxiety in myocardial infarction patients in the intermediate cardiac care unit', *Intensive Care Nursing*, **2**(2) 61–6.

Debelle, B. (1981), 'Relaxation and baby massage', *The Australian Nurses' Journal*, **1** 16–17.

Estabrooks, C. (1987) 'Touch in nursing practice, an historical perspective' *Journal of Nursing History*, **2**(2) 33–49.

Ernst, F. and Shaw, J. (1980) 'Touching is not taboo', *Geriatric Nursing*, **1**(5) 193-5.

Goodykoontz, L. (1979) 'Touch: attitudes and practice' *Nursing Forum*, **18**(1) 4-17.

Grad, B., Cadoret, R. and Paul, G. (1961) 'An unorthodox method of treatment on wound healing in mice' *International Journal of Parapsychology*, **3** 5–24.

Harrison, A. (1986) 'Getting the massage' *Nursing Times*, **82**(48) 24–5.

Hefferman, A. and Mott, S. (1984) 'Baby massage – a teaching model', *The Australian Nurses' Journal'*, **13**(6) 36–7.

Heidt, P. (1981) 'Effects of therapeutic touch on anxiety level of hospitalised patients' *Nursing Research*, **31** 32–7.

Hollinger, L. (1980) 'Perception of touch in the elderly', *Journal of Gerontological Nursing*, **6**(12) 741–6.

Holmes, P. (1986) 'Fringe benefits', in *Nursing Times*, **82** 20, 22.

Husband, L. (1988) 'Therapeutic touch: a basis for excellence', in Johnson, R. (ed.) *Recent Advances in Nursing. Excellence in Nursing*, Churchill Livingstone, Edinburgh.

Jackson, R. (1977) '*Massage Therapy: The Holistic Way to Physical and Mental Health*, Thorsons Publishing Group, Wellingborough.

Jackson, S. (1985) 'The touch process in rehabilitation', *The Australian Nurses' Journal*, **14**(11) 43-5.

Joachim, G. (1983b) 'The effects of two stress management techniques on feelings of well-being in patients with inflammatory bowel disease', *Nursing Papers*, **15**(4) 5–18.

Joachim, G. (1983a) 'Step-by-step massage techniques' *Canadian Nurse*, **4** 32–5.

Johnson, B. (1965) 'The meaning of touch in nursing', *Nursing Outlook*, 13 59–60.

Kaufmann, M. A. (1964) ' Autonomic responses as related to nursing comfort measures', *Nursing Research*, **13**(1) 45–55.

Knable, J. (1981) 'Hand holding : one means of transcending barriers of communication', in *Heart-Lung*, **10**(6) 1106–11.

Krieger, D. (1975) 'The therapeutic touch: the imprimatur of nursing', *American Journal of Nursing*, **75**(5) 748–87.

Krieger, D. (1979) *The Therapeutic Touch: How to use your Hands to Help and Heal*, Prentice Hall, New Jersey.

Lader, M. and Matthews, A. (1970) 'Comparison of methods of relaxation using physiological measures', *Behavioural Research and Therapy Journal*, (8) 331–7.

Langland, R. M. and Panicucci, C. (1982) 'Effects of touch on communication with elderly confused patients', *Journal of Gerontological Nursing*, **8** 152–5.

Le May, A. (1986) 'The human connexion', *Nursing Times*, **82**(47) 28–30.

Le May, A. and Redfern, S. (1987) 'A study of non-verbal communication between nurses and elderly patients', in Fielding, P. (ed.) *Research in the Nursing Care of Elderly People*, John Wiley and Sons Ltd., Chichester.

Longworth J. (1982) 'Psychophysiological effects of slow stroke back massage in normotensive females', *Advances in Nursing Science'*, **4**(4), 44–61.

Lorensen, M. (1983) 'Effects of touch in patients during a crisis situation in hospital', *Nursing Research: Ten Studies in Patient Care*, Wilson-Barnet (ed.), 179–92. John Wiley and Sons Ltd., Chichester.

Locsin, A. (1984) 'The concept of touch' *Philippine Journal of Nursing*, **54**(4), 114–23.

Mason, A. (1988) 'Massage', in Rankin-Box, D. (ed.), *Complementary Health Therapies: A Guide for Nurses and the Caring Professions*, Croom Helm, London.

McCorkle, R. (1974) 'Effects of touch on seriously ill patients' *Nursing Research*, **23** 125-32.

McNair, D. and Lorr, M. (1964) 'An analysis of mood in neurotics' *Journal of Abnormal Psychology*, **69** 620–7.

Melia, K. (1987) *Learning and Working: the Occupational Socialisation of Nurses*, Tavistock Publications Ltd., London.

Montagu, M. (1971) *Touching: The Human Significance of Skin*, Columbia University Press, New York.

Murphy, E. (1984) 'Practical management course, Module 15 ''High Touch'' techniques for managing the environment', *Nursing Management*, **15**(11) 79–81.

Naisbitt, J. (1982) *Megatrends*, Warner Brooks Inc., New York.

Pearson, A. and Vaughan, B. (1986) *Nursing Models for Practice*, Heinemann, London.

Pearson, A., Durand, I. and Punton, S. (1988) *Therapeutic Nursing: An Evaluation of an Experimental Nursing Unit in the British NHS*, Burford and Oxford Nursing Development Units, Oxford.

Preston, T. (1973) 'When words fail (Caring for the Aged)' *American Journal of Nursing*, 73 2064–6.

Quinn, J. (1984) 'Therapeutic touch as energy exchange: testing the theory', *Advances in Nursing Science*, **6**(2) 42–9.

Randolph, G. (1984) 'Therapeutic and physical touch: physiological response to stressful stimuli', *Nursing Research*, **33**(1) 33–6.

Rowlands, D. (1984) 'Therapeutic touch: its effects on the depressed elderly', *The Australian Nurses Journal*, **13**(11) 45–52.

Seaman, L. (1982) 'Affective nursing touch', *Geriatric Nursing*, **3**(3) 162–4.

Sims, S. (1986a) 'The effects of slow-stroke back massage on the perceived well-being of female patients receiving radiotherapy for cancer', MSc thesis in nursing, Kings College, University of London.

Sims, S. (1986b) 'Slow stroke back massage for cancer patients', *Nursing Times*, Occasional Paper, **82**(13) 47–50.

Turton, P. (1988) 'Healing: therapeutic touch', in Rankin-Box, D. (ed.) *Complementary Health Therapies: A Guide for Nurses and the Caring Professions*, Croom Helm, London.

Turton, P. (1989) 'Touch me, feel me, heal me', *Nursing Times*, **85**(19) 42–4.

Tutton, E. (1987) 'The effect of slow-stroke back massage on the perceived well-being of elderly female patients in a nursing unit', MSc thesis in nursing, Kings College, University of London.

Watson, W.H. (1975) 'The meanings of touch: geriatric nursing', *Journal of Communication*, **25** 104–10.

Wharton, A., Pearson, A. (1988) 'Nursing and intimate physical care: the key to therapeutic nursing', in Pearson, A. (ed.) *Primary Nursing: Nursing in the Burford and Oxford Nursing Development Unit*, Croom Helm, London.

Wise, R. (1989) 'Flower power', *Nursing Times*, **85**(22) 45–7.

Chapter 8

Breaking the mould: a humanistic approach to nursing practice

CHRISTINE MCKEE

THE SCIENTIFIC METHOD

During the Dark and Middle Ages, people held a different attitude towards knowledge. They believed first, that only a privileged few were entitled to have knowledge; second that all knowledge of any importance had already been acquired by the Greeks. For example, to learn about bees, one didn't observe bees – instead, one went to the manuscripts to read what the ancients had written about them.

Eventually a thaw occurred, which we know as the Renaissance (which means 'rebirth'). The prevailing attitudes were overthrown. Pioneering men like Francis Bacon taught that all knowledge had not been acquired. Everywhere there was renewed excitement as men observed Nature to discover her secrets for themselves. (Bacon himself died of pneumonia, contracted after he buried a dead chicken in the snow to discover if it would be preserved.)

One of Bacon's legacies to us was a systematic method of acquiring knowledge, which we today call the scientific method and which is a system of experimentation used to discover natural laws. An important part of the scientific method is the notion of 'determinism' – that is, if the same experiment is performed under the same conditions, the same outcome will be observed time after time. For many centuries scientists believed that determinism itself was a law of nature, i.e. given an adequate understanding of the initial conditions and all the mechanisms involved, an outcome could always be predicted. In other words, Nature was essentially predictable.

Throughout the ensuing centuries science did indeed make many dramatic and impressive advances, based on the method. And as a consequence, many other disciplines jumped on the bandwagon and attempted to use its philosophies and methods to advance their own understanding. Nursing was one of them. The majority of present-day nursing theories are 'in the tradition of classical 17th century science' and, as such, 'maintain that a human being, like the universe, can be considered machine-like, orderly, predictable, observable and measurable' (Benner and Wrubel, 1989).

Application of the scientific method and its philosophies to nursing, however, has not seen the same success as have the physical sciences. One problem is that it tends to have a dehumanising effect on the process of nursing and encourages a fragmentation of the individual into parts and systems. Aggleton and Chalmers (1986) suggest that nurses criticise models such as these for being too mechanistic in their identification of human needs, 'dehumanising the process of nursing by drawing an analogy between a human being and a machine with parts and systems within it. . . '

A second problem is that this approach simply doesn't work! Benner (1985) seconds a statement made by Merleau Ponty which most health professionals already know from their own experience 'that no strictly bottom-up explanation – that is, explanation from the cellular level up to the lived experience of health and illness – can adequately explain or accurately predict the particular course of an illness, nor can it explain the maintenance of health. We know that laboratory data frequently do not match the illness experience. People do not die or survive strictly according to our best biochemical or physiological accounts'.

It is interesting to note, after this, that even in the physical sciences the scientific method and determinism were never totally successful. Finally, in the 1920s workers in the new field of Quantum Mechanics actually proved what some scientists had begun to suspect for some time: namely, that determinism is not a law of nature. Specifically, scientists who were attempting to predict the position and motion of the electron in its orbit around the atom's nucleus, found that it could never be done. Motion within the atom, fundamental building block of the universe, is governed by probability. The world we live in is not totally predictable, after all.

HUMANISM AND NURSING

In the 1960s and 1970s humanistic nursing which was more consistent with the new thinking in science, began to emerge. Humanistic nursing is not exactly a theory of nursing, but more an approach which treats the human being as unique and unpredictable, which attempts to view him as a whole, with emphasis on his own perspective of the lived experience.

Perhaps the best known exponents of humanistic nursing are Josephine G. Paterson and Loretta T. Zderad (1976) who put forward a humanistic method of nursing which is based on a blend of existential and phenomenological ideas. They propose that nurses 'consciously and deliberately approach nursing as an existential experience'. What follows is largely an exploration of the Paterson and Zderad formulation.

An understanding of Existentialism is fundamental to humanistic nursing. It is a complex philosophy. 'By its very nature, existentialism is not a system and there are, in fact, almost as many existentialisms as there are existentialist philosophers' (Clemence 1966).

Fundamentally, however, existentialism is the study of existence, and the term 'derives from the Latin verb 'existere', which means to stand out from, emerge or become. Existence is therefore emergent; it is a process of coming into being, or becoming, rather than a state of being' (Graham, 1986). And while there are many different variations of the philosophy, certain important themes run throughout:

1. As above, the belief that man's existence is not a state of being, rather it is a process of becoming.
2. The belief that man makes himself, through the courageous and honest use of freedom in the face of situation limits such as illness, grief, anxiety and solitude (Clemence 1966).
3. A belief in man's freedom, choice and personal responsibility.
4. Sadly, that aloneness is a fundamental condition of life. The individual nature of our experiences traps us within our own separate realities which we are never able to penetrate or communicate completely.
5. Therefore that determinism and, in particular, human predictability, must be rejected. How can one predict what one can't fully understand?

6. The belief that life and others are to be studied from within out. 'For the existentialist the particular is seen from within, from the view of the lived life' (Gulino, 1982).
7. A wariness of groups, classes, categories. A distrust of abstractions.
8. The use of phenomenology to study being.

From an existentialist perspective, human beings are unique and unpredictable, and a major thrust of humanistic nursing is to view the individual as a whole, with emphasis on the individual's own perspective. These are perhaps the key differences between humanistic nursing and other modes of thought guiding nursing theory, such as systems, developmental and symbolic interactionist theories, which are closely linked to the scientific method, and, as such, are deterministic. Pearson and Vaughan (1986) state that symbolic interaction (threads of which can be seen in most nursing models), drawn to its logical conclusion, suggest that responses to a given situation can be predicted. Therefore, trial and error behaviours are ultimately unnecessary. Likewise, developmental theory centres around growth and change which occurs in recognised stages and is caused by identifiable variables and moves in a predictable direction (Pearson and Vaughan, 1986).

Indeed, Graham (1986) points out the irony in the fact that 'at the very time scientists were awakening to the possibility [that man is] more akin to cosmic consciousness than a machine, psychology, in its insistence on so-called 'objective' fact, was rejecting all subjective phenomena as unscientific'. Quoting Koestler, she continues:

'Materialism is 'vieu jeux' a century out of date. Only you psychologists still believe in it. It is a funny situation. We know that the behaviour of an electron is not completely determined by the laws of physics. You believe that the behaviour of a human being is completely determined by the laws of physics. Electrons are unpredictable, people are predictable. And you call this psychology.'

To borrow again from scientific thought: physicists say there are certain absolutes like the speed of light and the absolute zero in temperature which can never be achieved – but can be approached ever more closely. Likewise in humanism, it is not possible to understand another individual completely. And yet is is possible to approach a complete understanding ever more closely. The method they advocate is phenomenology.

To begin with, phenomena can be defined as any object or occurrences perceived by the senses. Scientists are quick to acknowledge that objective science has difficulty treating the elements of our experience which are not readily quantifiable. The language of positivistic science is too impoverished, say Benner and Wrubel (1989), to give an adequate account of the occurrences in everyday life. Phenomenology seeks to redress the balance by attempting to study all aspects of our experience. It is concerned with how it feels to be a certain person in a certain situation.

Just how phenomenology attempts this is a matter for much study. Hilgard et al. (1979) describe the phenomenological method of enquiry as a focus on subjective experience, which is not concerned with prediction and control, but with understanding the individual's inner life and experiences.

Husserl, the father of phenomenology, was 'committed to the clarification of experience and its objects' (Graham 1986). To that end he put forward a phenomenological method comprising three main phases:

1. Intuition (with a focus on the phenomenon of consciousness);
2. Discovery of the various constituents of such phenomena and their relationships;
3. Description or communication of these perceptions.

Maslow (1968) maintained that 'existentialism rests on phenomenology, i.e. it uses personal subjective experience as the foundation upon which abstract knowledge is built'.

APPLICATIONS

Having gained a broad understanding of the philosophy behind humanistic nursing, let us look in more detail at how Paterson and Zderad see its practice.

Paterson and Zderad (1976) describe the humanistic approach to nursing practice as a 'system, mode of thought or action in which human interests, values, and dignity are taken to be of primary importance'. The object of humanistic nursing, they say, is to view the individual as a whole rather than as a series of problems to be solved, with emphasis on the individual's own perspective of the lived experience.

They endorse the theme from existentialism, that man is free to choose and to become through his own choice – that we are ultimately responsible for what happens in our lives. Hence health is described as becoming all that is humanly possible. Nursing aims to develop human potential to its upmost: its goal is well-being and more-being.

Paterson and Zderad see nursing as the nurturing response of one person to another in need. They urge the nurse to be with the patient in the fullest sense, which requires turning one's attention towards the patient and communicating one's availability. Rather than asking the nurse 'What did you do?' in a nurse-patient situation, one might ask 'What happened between you?'

In order to be completely effective in this way, the nurse must herself approach nursing as an existential experience. Nursing is itself a lived experience, a response to a human situation which the nurse shares with another. It involves a transactional relationship, the meaningfulness of which requires that the nurse have a conceptual awareness of self and an acceptance of the uniqueness and value of the other.

The humanistic nurse will also appreciate the differences between our own angular views of the world. She will accept that man's differences are 'realities that are beyond the negative-positive good-evil standard of judgement' Peterson and Zderad (1976):

> 'Nursing is concerned with how this particular man, with his particular history, experiences being labeled with this general diagnosis and being admitted, discharged, and living out his life with his condition as he views it in-his-world.'

For the humanistic nurse existential awareness requires an authenticity with oneself. An in-touchness with who we are, the sensations we experience, our responses, awareness of our potential, are all reflected in our relationships with others. The more open to ourselves we are, the less of ourselves we have to exclude, the more we can be open with and share with others. 'This quality of personal authenticity allows one's responsible chosen actions to be based in human knowledge rather than human defensiveness' (1976).

This approach to nursing has to be personally invested in. It can't be superimposed on a nurse from the outside by another. In a spatial sense, a nurse can be ordered into a parallel existence with another. But 'being existentially and genuinely present with another is different' (1976).

Nursing, then, is viewed as a lived dialogue, 'a lived human act', which occurs within the domain of health and illness. Paterson and Zderad (1976) see it as comprising actions: meeting; relating; presence; call and response.

Meeting

At the first meeting, the patient and the nurse each bring their own set of goals and expectations. They both share the implicit expectation that the nurse will be helpful and that the patient needs assistance. Beyond that, each is a unique individual bringing all that he or she is or is not and, if the meeting is planned, each comes with feelings of anticipation, anxiety, dread, hope, fear, pleasure, impatience, hostility, dependence, responsibility. Each has a choice of openness, and each may have a different view of the precise need and the kind of help required.

In addition, the nurse may have prior knowledge of the patient and may bring preconceived ideas.

Relating

From a humanistic nursing perspective, two relationships are considered essential to the clinical nursing process. Firstly, the subject-object, 'I-it' relationship: although it is possible and sometimes necessary to observe the patient objectively, the person as object 'can make himself knowable or set up barriers to objectification. He can keep his thoughts to himself, remain silent or deliberately conceal some of his qualities' (1976).

Secondly, the subject-subject, 'I-Thou' relationship: through this relationship 'it is possible to know a person in his individuality' (1976).

Presence

Presence involves being with the patient in the fullest sense, being open and available. The nurse may be attentive but refuse to give of him or herself. Actions may not necessarily signify presence, but presence can be revealed directly and unmistakably in a glance, touch or tone of voice. Contained within genuine dialogue is a quality of unpredictability or spontaneity. For genuine dialogue to occur, there must be openness, receptivity and availability. 'The open or available person reveals himself as "present"' (1976).

Call and response

Call and response are transactional: the patient calls for help, the nurse responds. The nurse calls for the patient's participation, and the patient responds.

The patient's call may be non-verbal, and may be indicated by posture, colour or facial expression. The nurse's response is influenced by the value he or she places on time, place and agency policy, also on the patient's independence, motivation, rehabilitation, growth and strengths. 'Our interpretations of the patient's calls as well as our responses are colored by the aim of our practice' (1976).

Consistent with the above theory, Paterson and Zderad give no clear guidance concerning a goal-directed nursing care plan. The 'goal', as already stated, is the well-being and more-being of the patient. Furthermore, the ability and willingness to be with another in the fullest sense 'cannot be superimposed on a nurse clinician . . . . It must be personally and responsibly chosen and invested in.' The philosophy behind a care plan is also a subtle endorsement of determinism and predictability, which humanism rejects.

In general, the Paterson and Zderad methodology moves away from a positivist problem-solving approach, as the goals of phenomenology are diametrically opposed to those of a positivist epistemology of practice.

'Phenomenology seeks attestation of the meaning of a situation to a participant. Positivism seeks general objective categories within the universal. Phenomenology prizes differences, variations, and struggles for their representation as parts of the whole.' (Paterson and Zderad 1976)

Attempting to divide the patient into a list of problems, the nurse may lose sight of the complex relationships between those problems, which are often as important as the problems themselves. We can draw an analogy here with the protein molecule, which is a long chain of amino acids. But what gives the protein molecule its ability to function is its unique and characteristic shape it assumes as the chain folds back on itself many times to form a compact, ball-like arrangement. It is the shape which allows the protein molecule to interact with just the right other molecules in just the right way (lock and key mechanism) to perform its function as an enzyme in the body.

An effort to string out the protein molecule in order to itemise its component amino acids denatures the protein so that, having lost the shape that it depended on, one can no longer understand how it functions. Likewise, an attempt to characterise the patient as a list of problems can lead to only a partial understanding of his situation.

The argument against the positivistic approach finds a second voice in Donald Schon (1983). Schon suggests that practitioners who do use the positivistic approach may respond to complex situations by cutting the situation to fit professional knowledge, and by forcing situations into a mould through selectively ignoring data which fall outside, by attributing failure to personality, or disregarding problem clients by labelling them. Schon sees this forcing of practice situations into moulds as being inherent in a problem-solving approach. On the other hand, if we allow the uniqueness of the patient to shine through with all his complexities left intact, perhaps this could be avoided.

Schon suggests that a positivist epistemology of practice rests upon three principles:

1. the separation of means from ends;
2. the separation of research from practice;
3. the separation of knowing from doing.˙

However, in the real world these dichotomies do not hold, and Schon forwards the notion of 'reflection in action' as a description of what actually happens in practice. It may be described as a conversation with the situation, during which practitioners will reflect on intuitive understandings of the phenomena which are derived from their own repertoire of familiar examples and themes. Using this approach, ideas are exchanged backwards and forwards, means and ends are framed interdependently, knowing and doing are inseparable. The practitioner will use his repertoire of knowledge, theory and past experiences in responding to the patient's uniqueness. Schon talks about 'cutting the situation to fit professional knowledge'. Nurses who follow a problem-solving approach may find themselves narrowing their field of vision to take in only the problems which look as though they can be solved – and stepping over the ones which don't appear solvable. Moreover, the nurse who is orientated towards solving, curing, doing, will feel helpless in the face of situations where he or she doesn't know what to do when, in fact, perhaps 'doing' is not called for, but merely being with and understanding.

Humanistic nursing, on the other hand, is far less limiting because the nurse isn't trying to solve problems. Instead, his or her aim is to understand and to be with the patient – to explore the situation so that both nurse and patient may reach a deeper understanding. Perhaps this understanding may lead to a resolution of some sort – possibly a solution even, or an acceptance, or an awareness. But in all cases the question is not 'What did you do?', but 'What happened between you?'

To say that a care plan is not appropriate, however, is not to say that the care should not be well documented. Paterson and Zderad advocate a phenomenological approach to describe the lived nursing experience, and are quite explicit as to how it should be done: 'Severe self-discipline enters into describing nursing experience with the rigor of how it was lived'. In describing the nursing experience, the humanistic nurse will carefully record what she comes to know, that is, the knowable responses of the individual being nursed, the nurse's own observations and responses, and also her experiences as a participant. The nursing record may in part take the form of a journal. However, it will bear little relation to the nursing record known as the 'kardex' or 'kalamazoo', which all too frequently is 'let fall to mediocre common forms' (Paterson and Zderad 1976).

As stated earlier, Paterson and Zderad's phenomenological approach requires attitudes of openness and awareness. It involves getting in touch with one's sensations and feelings, and it allows for an intuitive grasp of the situation. As a methodological process, the phenomenological approach is subjective-objective and intuitive-analytic, that is, 'being with' (subjective, intuitive, knowing and experiencing) and 'looking at' (objective, analysing).

Paterson and Zderad describe five phases in their methodology, which they call the Phases of Phenomenologic Nursology, and which are as follows:

1. preparation for the nurse knower coming to know;
2. nurse knowing the other intuitively;
3. nurse knowing the other scientifically;
4. nurse complementarily synthesising known others;
5. succession within the nurse from the many to the para-doxical one.

George (1985) has compared these stages to the assessment, analysis, data collection and diagnosis stages of the nursing process. It is perhaps important to repeat at this point, however, that whereas the planning phase of the nursing process describes a goal or outcome to be reached by the patient and that specific nurse actions are clearly spelled out in detail, the phenomenological method 'does not describe the formation of a goal-directed nursing care plan. Humanistic nursing is concerned with being with another who is in need. The goal of more-being or well-being is accomplished through dialogue' (George, 1985).

ASSESSMENT USING THE FIVE PHASES OF
HUMANISTIC NURSING

Preparation for the nurse knower coming to know

This first phase in the methodology can be described as a process of preparing the mind and becoming aware of one's own values.

Paterson and Zderad (1976) tell us that in order to be open to the data of experience using a phenomenological approach, one must strive to eliminate that which exists in the mind prior to and independent of the experience, holding in abeyance theoretical presuppositions, interpretations, labels and judgements. Likewise, they remind us that thhe nurse's experience of his or her lived world may be dulled by habituation. In order to be open and receptive to the data, the nurse must prepare herself psychologically for a new experience – she must 'break through the tunnel vision of routine' (1976).

Nurse knowing the other intuitively

This phase can be seen as the beginning of assessment, a taking in of the nursed's whole experience all at once. George (1986) equates this phase with the pre-assessment phase of the nursing process.

For the humanistic nurse, the use of intuition is an important part of the overall assessment. The nurse's all-at-once grasp of the nursed's whole experience or his or her overall impression of the situation will likely occur at the initial contact with the patient.

Nurse knowing the other scientifically

In this phase, there is a forward movement from intuition to analysis. Data is collected, mulled over, analysed, sorted out, compared, contrasted and interpreted.

Following the nurse's intuitive experience of the other, she conceptualises it in accordance with her own human potential. This involves using words which Paterson and Zderad define as known symbols and categories to convey the experience. They make the point that whilst 'our actual experienced lived worlds flow in an all-at-once fashion', humanly we can only express the experience sequentially. George (1985) compares this to the assessment and early analysis phase of the nursing process.

Nurse complementarily synthesising known others

During this phase, the nurse examines the data and experience of the nursed in the light of scientific and previous knowledge – comparing, contrasting and synthesising to an expanded view, and considering the relationships between the phenomena.

Succession within the nurse from the many to the paradoxical one

During this phase, a conclusion is reached and the nurse comes up with a 'conception or abstraction which is an expression of the investigator in her here and now' (1976).

According to existentialist philosophy, it is impossible for one individual to know another completely, but it is possible to approach an understanding. Phase five, then, represents a breakthrough which Paterson and Zderad hope will occur in the nurse's understanding, having synthesised the data and nursed's experience with 'known others' – i.e. having brought together everything which she has learned about this patient and other patients, and examined it in the light of known theory and previous experience.

Formulation of a diagnosis or patient problem was not intended. However, George (1985) does compare this stage to the diagnosis stage of the nursing process. It must be borne in mind, though, that the conclusion reached will be broader than the classifications, and will reflect a synthesis of the data and the interrelatedness of the phenomena experienced by the patient.

A CASE STUDY

To help make the above discussion more concrete, and as a practical example of the assessment process from a phenomenological perspective, we might consider Laura, a 57-year-old woman diagnosed as having inoperable carcinoma of the stomach. She was in the terminal stages of her illness and was being cared for at home by her husband with the help of the district nurses. Before I visited Laura, she was described to me as neurotic, highly anxious, demanding and difficult. My preparation for 'coming to know' included clearing my mind of preconceived stereotyped ideas about her prior to the first visit, in order that I might be open and receptive to what this illness experience might mean to her.

Coming to know Laura intuitively began for me with the initial visit. During our first meeting, Laura appeared to be open, friendly, and willing to talk. She stated that she knew she was dying, and appeared to have a philosophical attitude towards death. Laura described her relationship with her husband as very close and loving. At face value, she appeared to be well in control of her situation, fully accepting of death, and stating that she felt no anger. However, intuitively I felt that she was holding a lot back. She was too bright and cheerful, too willing to talk about a very deep subject on a rather superficial level to a complete stranger. She had a pinched facial expression, and her smile appeared forced. Laura was a very articulate lady – interesting and easy to talk to. She had been a teacher prior to her illness and had had books published. So had her husband. I felt that it was extremely important to her that she remain in control.

Coming to know Laura scientifically began with the collection of the initial data. Data collection took place over a four-day period following my first visit, and consisted of biographical data, history of present illness and hospital admissions, physical assessment, pain assessment which also included assessment of psychological state, self-concept, relationships, spiritual well-being, attitude to dying, domestic background, hobbies/interests and medications.

Over the course of the assessment, inconsistencies appeared which suggested a discrepancy between Laura's statement of her calm acceptance and her actual behaviour, reinforcing my earlier intuition. For example:

1. Although Laura worried about her husband having too much to do, she persisted in finding him things to do which would keep him near her, but which did also greatly increase his workload.
2. Laura insisted that minor building work on the house be carried out, even though her husband felt it was unnecessary and only served to increase the level of stress which he experienced.
3. She was obsessional about detail, and had to supervise carefully all physical tasks performed for herself and in the household. (She would never allow the nurses to fill the washbowl with water, for instance.)

Complementarily synthesising the facts gathered required examining the assessment data and Laura's experience in the light of known theory and my own previous experience. Among the known theory I considered were the findings of

McIntire and Cioppa (1984), who remind us that 'typically a person with cancer has little or no control over the course of the disease'; Fitzgerald (1983), who notes that the greater the individual's expectation of control, the greater the perceived powerlessness if the patient does not indeed have control (we might remember that I thought Laura's expectation of control was high); and Twycross (1978), who reminds us that a person's pain threshold will vary according to mood and morale. Therefore, attention must be paid 'to factors that modulate pain threshold such as anxiety, depression, and fatigue'.

It is important to point out that although the collection of data and the full analysis of the nursing situation took place over a four-day period, the implementation of nursing care had obviously begun at the first visit. One can say that a much clearer picture was established by the fourth day of initial assessment, however, and that intellectually the first four phases occur very quickly in order to implement much-needed care. One can almost say that the nurse goes through the first four phases many times: once to implement initial care, then again to arrive at the expanded view which occurs during phase five, and then many more times as the situation is re-assessed, the nurse-patient relationship develops and deepens, and fresh break-throughs in understanding occur.

Having looked at the patient intuitively, collected assessment data, and analysed it in the light of known theory and past experiences, the nurse enters phase five, which consists of a breakthrough in her understanding of what this person is experiencing at this moment in time. She does not, however, list the patient's problems. Rather, she views them as an interrelated part of the whole experience. (See Figure 8.1.)

In Laura's case the leap in understanding came with the awareness that anxiety and fear made her more demanding, and that her feelings of loss of control further exacerbated the anxiety. Although she had admitted to the association between pain and some anxiety, she had not as yet admitted to fear. This leap was validated during the ensuing weeks.

Much of the care planned for Laura revolved around interventions to help reduce her feelings of powerlessness. It was thought that many of Laura's behaviour patterns demonstrated feelings of loss of control – for instance, her need

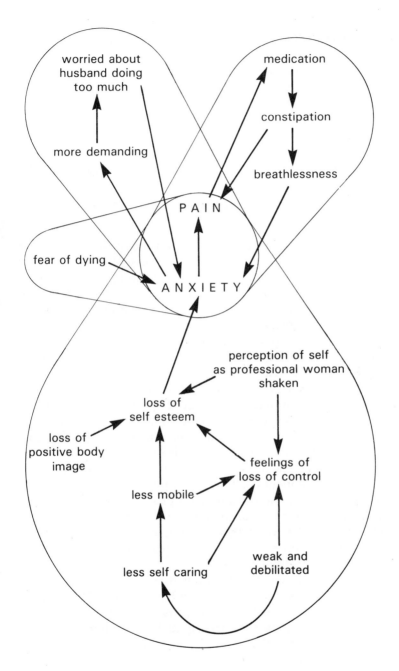

Figure 8.1

to keep strict control over the household activities, even though she knew her husband was perfectly able to cope, and that her constant worrying and niggling only added to his feelings of tension. Nursing measures put forward by McIntire and Cioppa (1984) to help reduce feelings of powerlessness include:

1. helping patients understand actions of drugs and goals of therapies;
2. discussion rationale for treatments;
3. exploring fears and fantasies associated with the cancer experience;
4. encouraging active participation in decision-making and care.

Enabling the patient to assume control over his or her own care experience is consistent with existential philosophy, which states a belief in man's freedom, choice and personal responsibility. Paterson and Zderad (1976) remind us that 'for the process of nursing to be truly humanistic it must bear out, that is, be a lived expression of, the nurse's recognition and valuing of nursing as an opportunity for the development of the human person.' Equally, they point out the importance of the nurse having the opportunity to experience for herself 'the growth-promoting character of responsible choosing' as she makes 'responsible competent professional judgments'. The nurse having had this experience will more readily recognise its value in the lives of others, and will be looking out for opportunities to encourage the patient to exercise his freedom of choice.

The humanistic nurse wants to provide the sort of climate in which the patient will have every opportunity to participate to the full in his own health care programme and therefore will 'nurture his human potential for responsible choosing' (1976). In order to do this, the nurse has to relinquish the authoritarian nurse role and surrender the decision-making authority to the patient.

It is naïve, however, to assume that all patients are willing and able to take on this new and unfamiliar role, and the humanistic nurse will need to consider ways in which she might help the patient to participate in his or her own health care programme. For example, she might look to Gadow (1981), who forwards the concept of existential advocacy. This differs from paternalism (i.e. making an 'assumption about what individuals should want to do') and from consumerism (i.e. 'protecting individuals' right to do what they want'), by helping the individual clarify his or her own values in the situation, enabling decisions to be reached which express the individual's 'reaffirmed, perhaps recreated, complex of values'. In this way the individual's decision is truly self-determined, instead of merely being 'a decision which is not determined by others'.

Gadow (1981) proposes this concept as a philosophical foundation upon which the patient and nurse freely decide the type of relationship they will have – for example parent and child, friend and friend, or colleague and colleague.

EVALUATION OF THE HUMANISTIC APPROACH TO NURSING PRACTICE

How appropriate is this method to most nursing situations?

We can respond by noting that the clinical area itself has little bearing on the effective use of the approach. Rather, the philosophy of the nursing staff is more likely to influence its success. For example, its use will be most effective:

1. When valuing the patient's personal choice takes precedence over strict nursing routines.
2. When ward organisation, for example primary nursing, allows for relationship building.
3. When nurses feel able to let go of the traditional authoritarian paternalistic nurse role.
4. When the individual nurse feels ready to invest in a deep commitment to the nurse-patient relationship. It cannot be stressed strongly enough that humanistic nursing cannot be imposed upon a nurse. Also that the nurse has a right to be honoured as a unique individual, as well, and that his or her differences should not be subjected to a positive-negative, good-evil, standard of judgement.
5. When all the nursing team are in harmony about the use of the approach. However, an individual nurse can incorporate many of the philosophies inherent in humanistic nursing practice into his or her own individual approach to patient care.
6. When the nurse's assessment skills are well developed.

Let us also point out that the above do not suggest actual weaknesses in humanistic nursing itself. Rather, they affirm that humanistic nursing cannot be imposed like a template on nursing practice. We might say, however, that they do imply limitations to the use of the theory, which requires special commitment and professional maturity.

On the other hand, there are some actual deficiencies in the method. One recognised by George (1985) is that it 'refers to the subjective interaction between two individuals and does not discuss the subjective encounter with a group of clients or with the family'.

This is borne out by my own experience. Establishing and maintaining a relationship with Laura tended to be all-consuming and, although support for her husband was considered, it was less heavily invested in. In retrospect this was seen to be a weak area in the planned care.

Also worthy of note is that humanistic nursing theory as described by Paterson and Zderad does not deal very comprehensively with physical care, and that this may be seen as a limitation in a general nursing setting.

As if in response, Paterson and Zderad recognise that caring for people's physical needs is one of nursing's basic concerns, but state that 'to view nursing from the perspective of the human situation, however, is to see beyond physical care, beyond the categorisation of man as a bio-psycho-social organism. The focus is on the person's unique being and becoming in his situation' (1976).

For example, by considering how the patient's world changes as his or her bodily functions change during illness, and how he or she experiences that world, the nurse will be aware that those things which he or she takes for granted such as 'hospital noises or odours, touching, bathing, feeding, sleep or meal schedules, may have very different meanings for individual patients. They may or may not be experienced at nurturing in a particular person's lived world' (1976).

Thus, the more basic concern within humanistic nursing practice will be the humanising or dehumanising effects of the nursing event. Humanistic nursing, therefore, is concerned with, but goes beyond, physical care in attempting to understand how each individual experiences his or her physical body within the context of both health and illness.

IMPLICATIONS FOR RESEARCH

The use of humanistic nursing has rich implications for research, as virtually every nursing situation can be a research situation. Humanism does not suffer the criticisms of a positivistic approach, that 'knowledge comes to be viewed as a product to be utilised', and that 'the role of the clinician in developing knowledge is overlooked' (Benner and Wrubel 1989). Schon states that a positivistic epistemology of practice separates research from practice – yet for many practitioners, practice is a kind of research . . . inquiry being a transaction with the situation in which knowing and doing are inseparable (Schon 1983).

Phenomenology was conceived by its founder, Husserl, as a 'scientific and exact method' for 'the clarification of experience and its objects' (Graham, 1986). Hilton (1987) describes phenomenology as one of the three schools of ethnography (the other two being ethnomethodology and interactionism) and, as such, an important component of ethnographic research.

The nurse using a phenomenological method will describe perceived nursing occurrences, and will be collecting data which is rich and meaningful, and which can reveal themes and patterns within similar nursing situations and provide a basis for further inquiry. The method is inductive, that is, it starts by gathering data and subsequently develops a hypothesis (as opposed to deductive, which starts with the hypothesis and then proceeds to test it). Thus it is a particularly useful method for exploring situations about which there is little current knowledge.

In short, nurses who use a phenomenological method for everyday nursing situations are researchers. Humanistic nursing, therefore, provides greater opportunity for the development of nursing knowledge to emerge from clinical practice, with the clinician being central to the process. Paterson and Zderad believe that compiling and complementarily synthesising phenomenological descriptions over time 'will build and make explicit a science of nursing' (1976).

SUMMARY

Once it was believed that the world is a great machine, and that it is only our imperfect understanding of how it works which keeps us from a certain knowledge of all things. When our understanding had advanced sufficiently, even human behaviour would be predictable.

Recently, however, science came to realise that it was more than our own imperfect understanding which bars the way. From the very atoms on upwards, uncertainty reigns. And few things in the universe – humans in particular – will ever be totally predictable.

Humanistic nursing is an approach to nursing which is sympathetic with this new outlook. It borrows the themes of existentialism and the methods of phenomenology, and suggests that:

1. The patient is more than a list of problems, more than the sum of his or her parts, and must be viewed as a whole. Efforts to use a machine as a model are doomed to only limited success.
2. The patient is alone in his experiences and is never completely knowable. He deserves our respect as a unique and unpredictable fellow being.
3. At the same time, nurses are human beings, too. To attempt to nurture and be with another human being as closely as possible requires that they approach nursing as an existential experience.
4. This requires openness and self-awareness before the necessary breakthroughs in understanding can occur. Professional maturity is called for. Nor is it an approach which can be successfully imposed from outside.
5. Because humanistic nursing is not a problem-solving exercise, the nurse is more free to bring her creativity to caring.
6. The transactions and the learning that can occur between two existential beings must largely be subjective. Phenomenology is often more appropriate than the tolls of objective science.
7. Finally, personal subjective experience is also 'the foundation upon which abstract knowledge is built', and therefore virtually every nursing situation is an opportunity for research. Compiling and synthesising phenomenological descriptions 'will build and make explicit a science of nursing'.

REFERENCES

Aggleton, P. and Chalmers, H. (1986) *Nursing Models and the Nursing Process*, Macmillan Publishers Ltd., London.

Benner, P. (1985) 'Quality of life: a phenomenological perspective on explanation, prediction, and understanding in nursing science', *Advances in Nursing Science* 8(1) 1–14.

Benner, P. and Wrubel, J. (1989) *The Primacy of Caring*, Addison-Wesley Publishing Company, Inc., California.

Clemence, Sr. M. (1966) 'Existentialism: a philosophy of commitment', *American Journal of Nursing*, 66(3) 500–5.

Fitzgerald, M.J. (1983) *Coping With Chronic Illness Overcoming Powerlessness*, F.A. Davis Co., Philadelphia.

Gadow, S. (1981) 'Existential advocacy: philosophical foundation of nursing', in Spicker, S.F. and Gadow, S. (eds) *Nursing: Images and Ideals Opening Dialogue With the Humanities*, Springer Publishing Company, New York.

George, J.B. (1985) *Nursing Theories: The Base for Professional Nursing Practice*, Prentice-Hall Inc., New Jersey.

Graham, H. (1986) *The Human Face of Psychology*, Open University Press, Milton Keynes.

Gulino, C.K. (1982) 'Entering the mysterious dimension of other: an existential approach to nursing care', *Nursing Outlook*, 30 352–7.

Hilgard, E.R., Atkinson, R.L. and Atkinson, R.C. (1979) *Introduction to Psychology*, (7th edn), Harcourt Brace Jovanovich Inc., San Diego.

Hilton, A. (1987) *Research Awareness Module 7: The Ethnographic Perspective*, Distance Learning Centre, South Bank Polytechnic, London.

Maslow, A.H. (1968) *Toward a Psychology of Being* (2nd edn), Van Nostrand Reinhold Company, New York.

McIntire, S.N. and Cioppa, A.L. (1984) *Cancer Nursing: A Developmental Approach*, John Wiley & Sons Inc., New York.

Paterson, J.G. and Zderad, L.T. (1976) *Humanistic Nursing*, John Wiley & Sons Inc., New York.

Pearson, A. and Vaughan, B. (1986) *Nursing Models for Practice*, Heinemann Professional Publishing Ltd., Oxford.

Schon, D.A. (1983) *The Reflective Practitioner*, Maurice Temple Smith Ltd., London.

Twycross, R.G. (1978) 'The assessment of pain in advanced cancer', *Journal of Medical Ethics*, 4 112–16.

Chapter 9

Taking up the challenge: the future for therapeutic nursing

ALAN PEARSON

INTRODUCTION

The preceding chapters have all, in some way, attempted to both define, explore and develop the concept of therapeutic nursing, and to describe pragmatically its performance in action. The purpose of this final chapter is somehow to bring all of this together and to outline some pointers for the future. The task is both daunting and exciting, for the future is something about which we dream, but not something which we can accurately predict. This chapter will set out some basic assumptions about therapeutic nursing; historically review the evolution of nursing as therapy; outline arguments which suggest that the therapeutic potential of nursing has been devalued and offer suggestions for the development of nursing as a therapeutic activity for the future.

THERAPEUTIC NURSING – BASIC ASSUMPTIONS

Lisbeth Hockey suggests that the term 'therapeutic nursing' has only recently been adopted, but that nursing has always possessed therapeutic potential and that Nightingale emphasised this without using the term specifically. Use of the term appears to have evolved from the work of Hall (1966), Tiffany (1977) and Alfano (1969). All three were cited by Pearson (1983) and their ideas were extensively developed in the establishment of Britain's first nursing development unit at Burford Community Hospital (Pearson 1985, 1988) and the subsequent setting up of the Oxford Nursing Development Unit. These ideas were developed further by McMahon (1988), Ersser (1988) and Muetzel (1988). The Burford initiative focused on Tiffany's notion of creating an environment where the nurse is the 'chief therapist', rather than the maintainer of order which enables other health workers to apply their therapies and on Alfano's assertion that the nurse who acts therapeutically '. . . sees her role not as an intervener or interpreter, but as a caring person and teacher'. Hall (1966) posited that nurses alone engage in intensely intimate activity in their professional role, and that this gives rise to opportunities for human closeness which can be used to therapeutic effect. Through concentrating on the notion that nursing as caring is a therapy in its own right, the Burford participants began to think and talk about therapy as a skilled, professional activity which has a positive effect on people in as much as it leads to the achievement of health or healing. This early thinking stemmed from Alfano's (1971) distinction between professional orientated nursing (or therapeutic nursing) and task orientated nursing (see Figure 9.1.)

The writings of early civilisations refer to nursing, and throughout the ages there appears to have always been a group of people engaged in nursing, although they were not always referred to as nurses. In the middle ages, nursing took on the cloak of altruism, and many of its practitioners (either religious men and women or knights) were the highly educated of society. Nineteenth-century reforms in nursing developed an opening for middle-class and working-class women to enter a workforce which was respectable, and which held out romanticised opportunities. In the 20th century, nursing has espoused the new religion of science and taken on the trappings of functionalism and objectivity.

NURSING AS CARING

Throughout all of this however, nurses and the communities they served have been cognisant, to a greater or lesser degree, of the core of nursing – the provision of care or nurturance. Pratt (1980) says that:

> 'Caring has an ancient lineage in nursing. It is impossible to review the history of the profession without finding the words used snynonymously. From the nurses of the ancient Hindu health care team (patient, nurse, doctor and drugs) and Hippocrates' students practising patient-centred problem-solving care, from the deaconesses and the Roman

Task orientated nursing	Therapeutic nursing
1. Looks upon intimate bodily care as a measure to produce comfort and modifies in the light of disease processes. Therefore, delegates majority of tasks related to intimate bodily care to staff who are least prepared to use closeness in teaching, learning situation. May or may not supervise staff engaged in these tasks. Gives intimate bodily care only to sickest.	1. Looks upon the comforting component of intimate bodily care and the closeness this engenders as an opportunity for nurturing i.e. fostering growth, healing, learning and modifies in relation to patient's concerns, feelings, as well as pathology. Therefore, performs all comforting measures related to intimate bodily care – delegates only work with things to nonprofessional staff thus freeing nurses to work with people.
2. Utilises other staff as substitute for nurse e.g. practical nurse, nursing auxiliaries etc.	2. Uses assistance of non-professional staff (messenger attendants who work with things) while professional nurse is working directly with patient, taking total responsibility for the nursing care involved with a group (i.e. maximum of eight patients).
3. Other therapists (e.g. physiotherapist) give their care directly to patients. Nurse acts as organiser.	3. Other therapists (e.g. physiotherapists) act as resource people to nurses in majority of situations – give direct care only when it is appropriate to nursing and calls for their most distinctive area of practice. Nurse acts as a 'final effector'. Nurse incorporates suggestions by other therapists in her daily nursing care.
4. Record-keeping emphasises clinical observations and symptoms and nursing tasks completed.	
5. Concerned with immediate treatment, less concentration on past and future continuity of care.	
6. Care organised around completion of assigned tasks and routines as applied to specific disease entity and organisation of services – may or may not be modified for patient.	4. Recording includes clinical observations and symptoms in relation to patients' activities, feelings and behaviour.
7. Major emphasis of care upon medications, treatment and assisting doctor.	

Figure 9.1 Task orientated nursing and therapeutic nursing (adapted from Alfano 1971).

8. Preventive care primarily concerned with:
   (a) preventing spread of infection;
   (b) prevention of further infection;
   (c) prevention of complications;
   (d) recurrence.
9. Often sees families and visitors as interfering with work, even during visiting hours.
10. Supports patient's expression of helplessness with comparative examples of others who have succeeded, or who have greater handicaps. Sets limits and restrictions upon patient.
11. Assignments divided by tasks with professional nurse predominantly involved in giving medications and performing 'more complex' treatments on an eight hour shift basis. Other tasks, many with patients, allocated to non-professional staff.
12. Atmosphere: hurried, pressured, emphasis upon importance of time, patient identified as 'one of many'.
13. Opportunities for patient and family teaching limited. Lip service with little follow-up.
14. Quality of teaching mostly explanation, orientation, fact giving – not conducive to learning (change of behaviour) since primarily done at readiness of nurse rather than patient. (Since non-professional nursing

5. Concerned with past history, future plans, and plans with patients immediate treatments with relation to these.
6. Care organised around requests and concerns of patient-organisation of service and routines flexible in the light of the above. Modified in relation to specific disease entity.
7. Major emphasis of care upon patient's feelings, concerns, goals and assisting him or her family through medical therapy.
8. Preventive care concerned with:
   (a) preventing spread of infection;
   (b) prevention of further infection;
   (c) prevention of complications;
   (d) new illnesses or recurrence of present illness; includes case finding in patients' families and patients.
9. Invites family to participate in patient care as patient and family member are willing and ready.
10. Helps patient explore his expression and feelings of helplessness and come clear on his own self-image and concept, thereby helping him to clarify his own goals. Helps patient determine and set his own limits.
11. Assignments divided by census and care needed. Each professional nurse assumes responsibility for complete care of patients assigned on a 24-hour basis.

Figure 9.1 *continued*

staff spend more time with patients than professional staff, what little teaching is done is performed by non-professional staff.)

15. Goal of teaching – to get patient to fit into accepted patterns, not disturb the routine, to get work done, to get the patient to do what is best for him. Early discharge emphasised.

16. Interprets doctor and his orders to the patient.

17. Predominantly task orien-tated rather than patient-orientated. Acts as though she sees nursing as a series of tasks done 'to', 'for', or 'at' patient on a time schedule.

18. Gives emotional support and reassurance on the basis of her evaluation of patient's need rather than at his request. Tends to discourage patients from expressing negative or unaccept-able feelings; instead introduces 'hopeful truths' e.g. 'don't worry, think of how much better you'll feel later'.

19. Attempts to help patient get over his concerns by diver-ting him with reports of her own extraneous activities. (Brings outside in.)

20. Often sees and evaluates patient through the eyes of nonprofessional staff whom she supervises.

21. Places emphasis of care on evaluation of reality of patient's needs on objective medical data, rather than on

12. Atmosphere; unhurried; easy, emphasis upon care, patient considered as individual.

13. Opportunities for patient and family teaching unlimited.

14. Quality of teaching empha-sises listening and reflecting what patient does and says, so that he can when he is ready explore his concerns and utilise facts. This includes evaluation and follow-up.

15. Goal of teaching – to help patient increase and utilise his strengths and his knowledge to achieve his goals; practice, performance, and self-evaluation. Discharge based on readiness of patient.

16. Interprets patient and his concerns to doctor and helps patient directly approach doctor in discussing plan of care.

17. Predominantly patient concern-orientated. Acts as though she sees nursing as a process in which she engages 'with' the patient and family to foster growth, learning and healing. Essentially she deals with the total life processes in finding solu-tions to human problems.

18. Uses and teaches problem facing and solving approach and methods. Accepts patient's expressions of worry and negative feelings; reflects these as well as those 'hopeful truths' the patient identifies.

19. Helps patients face and explore his or her own con-cerns. (Brings inside out.)

Figure 9.1 *continued*

subjective feelings of patient, and withholds or grants help in relation to these 'realities'.

22. Has predetermined expectations for goals and behaviour of patients. Accepts or rejects to the extent that they are able to meet these expectations.

23. Primarily concerned with patient's safety rather than his or her concepts of 'self' and 'personal dignity'. Expects or assumes that the patient will adapt to the hospital system.

24. Expects polite, courteous and co-operative behaviour of patient – often behaves less well him or herself. Fails to introduce self or call patient by name.

25. Concerned with finding out about the patient learning to understand and know him or her, gathering data, identifying the problem (increasing emphasis on nursing diagnosis and nursing care plans).

26. Sets goals and makes decisions for patient.

27. Fragmentation of care is more apt to be practised.

28. Receives direction often initiated by nursing supervisors.

29. Surrogate of doctor and other paramedical disciplines.

30. Participates as lesser member in team conference.

20. Sees patients through his or her own eyes and validates observations with peers, identifies his or her own feelings, and helps the patient evaluate him or herself. Involves members of the family whenever possible.

21. Places emphasis of care on expressed concerns and self-discovered needs and feelings which patient accepts as reality. Gives help in relation to above.

22. Accepts patient where he or she is and is willing to struggle with him or her in an attempt to find his or her way toward his or her own expectations.

23. In the absence of a 'hospital system' adjusts programme to the patient. Concerned with patient's 'concept of self' and his or her personal worth, as well as safety.

24. Allows patient to behave as he or she wishes short of physically hurting him or herself or others.

25. Concerned with giving patient opportunity to find out about and understand him or herself. He or she identifies the problem, decreasing emphasis on nursing diagnosis and nursing care plans – increasing emphasis on self-awareness and patient's plans.

26. Patients set goals and make decisions – nurses facilitate the process.

27. Integration of care is more likely to be produced.

28. May request and has available to him or her guidance and counselling from senior nurse.

Figure 9.1 *continued*

31. Channels contacts with community and family members through hospital-designated authorities – may or may not be nursing.
32. Records on special section of chart.
33. Wears uniform.
34. Cannot act any differently than he or she feels, regardless of appropriateness to nursing care situation.
35. Staffing patterns make necessary a concentration of nursing care during shift. Preponderance of nursing staff assigned to day hours; evening shift considered a relief shift for emergency and urgent care only.
36. Nursing practice discussed and evaluated in order to improve nursing service.
37. Victim of an authoritarian system which demands authoritative care.

29. Chief therapist, works with MD and other ancillary disciplines. Surrogate of patient.
30. Participates as leader in team conference.
31. Makes direct contact with community and family members.
32. Records on major part of record patient's progress notes with other disciplines.
33. Wears uniform or not depending upon his or her own wishes.
34. Grows in self knowledge and self awareness and as he or she learns is able to vary his or her behaviour appropriately to nursing care situation.
35. Staffing patterns organised so that same number of nurses assigned to evenings as to days; nursing care therefore able to be extended throughout day and evening hours.
36. Nursing practice analysed as a basis for synthesis of improved practice
37. Participant in liberating system which fosters democratic care.

Figure 9.1 *continued*

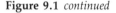

matrons of early Christianity, from the middle ages with its monks and nuns, its military Knights Hospitallers of St John and numerous other knights who were nurses, and the secular nursing orders, through the Renaissance in to the new world, through to the much maligned Mrs Gamp, through to Nightingale.'

Caring in this context was seen as a therapeutic activity which led to growth and healing.

The nature of caring

Whilst nurses can never claim to be the only health professionals who care, they can claim to be the only group whose central concern is that of human caring *per se*. Care and caring are complex concepts which beg for further exploration, yet are frequently seen as ordinary, simple and easy to put into practice.

Dunlop (1986) in her article 'Is a science of caring possible?', suggests that care can be interpreted as a deep involvement and engagement in the world which is central and necessary to any human activity. Care is seen as a global, human concept in which the care for things (concern) and caring for others (solicitude) makes human existence meaningful. Care has the same root as the word compassion, both deriving from the Celtic word 'cari' meaning 'to cry out with, to enter into the suffering'. The words care and compassion, then, are exactly the same. Commenting on this common meaning of care and compassion, Nouwen (1980) asserts that nurses should see care as their central mission, and says, that 'Out of care, cure can be born . . . Care broadens your vision; care makes you see around you; care makes you aware of possibilities'.

True caring is based on an attitude of nurturing – of helping another to grow. For the purposes of this chapter then, in referring to care or caring I am talking about this broad, global, human concept of investing oneself in the experience of another sufficiently enough to become a participant in that person's experience. This concept of caring absolutely demands an involved stance, and does not, according to Benner (1985):

' '. . . seek to control or master but to facilitate and uncover the possibilities inherent in the situation and the person. Caring provides empowerment' (not control). Indeed, 'technological self understanding causes a devaluation and misunderstanding of caring'.'

The need to place caring as a central concept in nursing has never been greater yet the caring components of nursing have become decentralised and are seen as the least sophisticated and subordinate to the therapeutic interventions of doctors and paramedical therapists.

The devaluing of nursing as caring

Nursing and caring as women's work

Throughout its history, nursing has fundamentally been concerned with human caring. Caring itself is also at the root of women's history. Whilst men have focused largely on the care and manipulation of the material world, women have always centred on the care of people in both their family environments and in their paid work.

Because of the prevalence of patriarchy and the over-whelming dominance of a masculine world view, human caring and its association with womanhood have persistently and consistently been both publicly devalued, yet privately desired. Colliere (1986) argues that, because of this, care is publicly invisible and that those who occupy themselves with it within the workforce are socially unconsidered, powerless and marginalised in terms of their perceived usefulness to society. Reverby (1987) explores this even further. In her exposé of nursing and caring as women's work, she highlights the dilemma of altruism (which is believed by the world to be the basis of nursing and caring) on the one hand, and autonomy (believed by the world to be the basis of rights and thus for the possession of legitimate power) on the other.

Colliere (1986) asserts that '. . . care remains invisible, priceless in health institutions as well as at home', whilst Reverby argues that caring is universally acknowledged as good and necessary, but that it is overly associated with altruism and in direct opposition to any notions of autonomy. She suggests that nurses need to 'create a new political understanding for the basis of caring and find ways to gain the power to implement it' . . . that nurses need '. . . power to practice altruism with autonomy'.

The development of nursing has been closely linked with the emergence of the women's movement, and its political position today is closely linked with the status of women and the dominance of the masculine world view. Ashley (1976) argues that nursing has been unable to occupy the strong power base in health care that it should have because of two interrelated factors:

1. Nursing is, and has been, a female dominated occupation and seen as legitimately 'women's work'.
2. The health care system in itself is paternalistic which has suppressed the development of nursing.

Whilst the status of individual and groups relates to a number of factors, gender is a significant issue in nursing's current and potential power base. As Vance *et al.* (1985) say:

'Feminist women and nurses have frequently experienced an uneasy relationship. Much of the energy in the women's movement has been directed toward moving into non-traditional fields of study and work. Nursing has been seen, therefore, as one of the ultimate female ghettos from which women should be encouraged to escape.'

There has been and still is a tendency for nursing, despite the rise in feminist thinking and activity, to espouse male values and to attempt to masculinise its practice and structures in order to gain power. Espousing masculine ideology and this appears to be the strategy for development in the latter half of this century.

In the UK, Nuttal (1983) reports that only 20% of registered nurses in 1983 were male, 43.8% of district nursing officers, and 50.5% of directors of nursing education were men. This may partly be a result of the limitations imposed on women by the community in terms of its prerequisites for promotion – unbroken records of employment, full-time commitment and putting work before all else. But it may also be partly due to nursing's rejection of feminist thinking and rationale. Has nursing quite deliberately pursued a masculine identity in order to achieve power in a male dominated world? Clay (1987) suggests that:

'The opposite view, of course, is that rather than imbuing a female profession with male values, we should be working to assert, develop and generate confidence in nursing's "femaleness".'

The apparent distance maintained between women nurses and the women's movement is therefore difficult to understand. This is especially so when one considers Mason and McCarthy's (1985) discussion on the politics of patient care.

Power in nursing, like power in general is thus exercised from a position of legitimacy, authority, professionalism and social unity.

Power and gender

Colliere suggests that because of the underestimation and devaluation of women, and therefore of care provided largely by women, nursing is part of a dominator-dominated system, where largely women nurses are dominated by largely male doctors and administrators. The powerlessness and subservience of nurses is seen therefore as directly attributable to sex or gender.

Game and Pringle (1983), in their description of the sexual division of labour in health care, argue that the symbolism of doctor/father, nurse/mother is the norm and that these lead to highly sexualised power relationships. They point out that women as the majority of health care providers (74.96%) are dominated by a male minority and that health care is characterised by obvious and ruthless sexism.

Because care is associated with women and women hold less power in society, it is shamefully devalued and has not until now been recognised as a subtle and powerful therapeutic force in health and healing.

THE FUTURE

A new era

Rogers (1983), in a paper titled 'Beyond the Horizon' and addressing the future of nursing, urges us:

> '. . . to glimpse a becoming, to see with that "third eye" . . . to speculate upon a dream and to watch that dream unfold . . . to create a new reality.'

A new era of nursing is now, I believe, in its beginnings. There have been gradual changes in world views held by society and nursing is beginning to demonstrate a shift away from its allegiance to a technical and task orientated view towards the adoption of new value stances.

Firstly nursing has espoused, or at least contemporary

rhetoric suggests so, the concept of holism as an intrinsic value. First described by Smuts in 1926, holism rests on two basic assumptions about people:

1. the individual always responds as a unified whole;
2. individuals as a whole are different from, and more than, the sum of their parts.

These basic assumptions espoused by nursing in the last 20 years indicate a movement away from the Cartesian ideas which demand that the person can be best understood by reducing her or him into her or his component parts.

Holism asserts that there is a need to study the whole being, including the manner in which the body and mind, for example, interact.

Secondly, nursing has espoused the philosophy of humanism. Often linked with the existentialist school of thought, humanism is based on the value of being human, of existing and of the quality of that existence.

Existentialism emphasises three main characteristics:

1. the uniqueness of the individual;
2. the importance of the meaning and purpose of human lives rather than truths about the whole universe and how it works;
3. the freedom of individuals to choose.

Humanistic existentialism asserts that there is a need to empower clients to make choices about the management of their own health. Bevis (1978) sees the embracing of these two views as '. . . the natural maturational philosophy for nursing'.

The espousing of holism and humanistic existentialism by nursing signals a major change in orientation, and is consistent with the responses in health care called for by such bodies as the World Health Organisation if 'Health for All by the Year 2000' is to become even partly realised.

Like nursing past, contemporary nursing is being influenced by and is responding to, emerging world views and the perceived needs of the consumers which these views generate.

Holism and humanism are becoming valued in society as a whole, which can be seen in changing attitudes to health and health care. For example there is an upsurge of interest in holistic health care and complementary therapies. Patients' associations and self-help groups are being established. Within nursing, corresponding efforts to promote patient autonomy and the right to make informed choices are becoming evident and partnership between nurses and clients (as opposed to being directive) are beginning to be seen as legitimate and valued. Nurses – and others – are now also beginning to realise that such an orientation actually 'makes a difference' to recovery rates and healing for clients . . . that nursing is a therapy as tangible and as effective as medical and paramedical therapies.

Since time immemorial, there has always been the assumption that nursing which has caring as a central concept, respects the person and is intensely human in nature, will assist people to maintain health, or to attain health when sick. For the past 100 years this has been superficially decentralised in understandings of the nursing role. As a result, nursing may have neglected to discover whether or not professional nursing which holds care, nurturance and humanness as a central concept actually does make a difference and if so, what it is about how nurses care which makes this difference. In other words is this sort of nursing therapeutic – does it attend to the healing process or help people attain or maintain health?

Evidence which supports the therapeutic potential of nursing

In this era of nursing, and our growing ability to articulate its nature, it would seem to be a feature of nursing activity, from the limited work done on exploring nursing and its effect on people, that it generally has a positive effect on people.

For example, patients cared for by nurse practitioners working within an in-patient rehabilitation setting compared favourably with physician-managed patients with six medical conditions (Weinberg *et al* 1983), MacCauley and Anderson's (1974) study of the nurse as a primary therapist with stroke patients describes a comparable degree of effectiveness when compared with team care, but at a significantly lower cost. Other studies by Sackett et al. (1977); Franklin (1974), Miller (1985) and Pearson (1985, 1987, 1988) all show that professional nursing has a therapeutic effect.

There is thus growing evidence that nursing is therapeutic and thus a strong enough basis for nurses justly to argue that the practice of nursing and the knowledge it stems from, and subsequently derives from it in action, should be valued and seen as a truly credible intervention to meet current and future health needs within our society. But this evidence is insufficent and there is still too little time and resources available for nursing to explore these issues.

In my own studies, nursing based on holistic and humanistic principles was the potent variable evaluated, and led to significant improvements in patient outcomes and to significant cost savings.

I am suggesting then, that from whence it came, modern nursing has passed through the three stages of development related to social relevance and reform described by Bevis (1978), and that it has seen a shift in world views which is leading it to a new era of nursing and that this is both grounded in nursing's past and desirable for meeting future societal needs for health care.

How do we get there?

Getting there easily and smoothly is dependent upon developing knowledge and new understandings about nursing and generating changes in practice which these new understandings demand, preparing future nurses to acquire abilities to enable them to view people holistically, and utilising political strategies to create a valuing of therapeutic nursing.

Developing new knowledge and changing practice

Nursing needs to invest more in its research endeavours into the therapeutic effects of its practice and to use these endeavours in a way which changes practice in reality. For the future, two major issues need to be pursued.

Firstly, nursing units devoted to the provision of nursing as the primary therapy need to be established more widely. This will serve a number of purposes. The creation of a nursing-centred environment will assert that nursing is indeed a therapy in its own right; develop knowledge through its actions, and provide a milieu for research and development. Such activity will enhance the ability of nursing to build up its own substantive base and to move practice in all settings towards a therapeutic orientation.

Secondly, research itself needs to be a much greater feature of initiatives which foster therapeutic nursing. Politically, hard, quantifiable data is needed to demonstrate that nursing does make a difference in terms of outcomes. More importantly, however, much of nursing is too sophisticated and complex to be studied from a stance which purports that the truth can only be exposed through the statistical analysis of quantifiable data. Other stances which see subjective and qualitative approaches to research as legitimate paths in seeking knowledge are closer to nursing's orientation and may well uncover much more than politically acceptable 'scientific' studies. Such approaches like nursing and caring, conflict with the hard, objective and masculine view of the world.

In developing new understandings and knowledge of nursing and in instituting desirable practice change, the setting up of nursing units and the pursuit of research utilising a range of methodological approaches is essential to the future of therapeutic nursing.

The preparation of future nurses

Education can play a pivotal role in supporting this new era of nursing. In terms of preparing future nurses, changes in nursing education offer considerable potential for empowering the new generation of nurses to meet future health needs. Higher education for nurses per se will not inevitably lead to positive development in itself, but the potential is most certainly there. The crucial variable lies in the design and offering of programmes which can best equip students with the categories of knowledge fundamental to the kind of nursing practice needed for the future.

Whilst the hospital schools may have been accused of an over-emphasis in the past on practice and nursing service and an under-emphasis on theoretical preparation, higher education may be accused in the future of an over-emphasis on theory and an under-emphasis on practice. In the drive to enhance nursing's theoretical underpinning, practice may be dismissed as non-theoretical and the fact that it is indeed a sophisticated intellectual pursuit which incorporates a variety of patterns of knowledge may be neglected. Education has both the capacity and responsibility to empower future nurses to draw on nursing's inheritance and to move forward into the emerging era of nursing by enabling students to acquire relevant categories of knowledge.

Building on nursing's past inheritance, contemporary nursing is, I believe, in an enviable position and is on the verge of what may be perhaps referred to as the emancipatory era of nursing. This era encompasses the context of a changing social relevance for nursing and changing world views and nursing education carries an awesome responsibility in supporting this era. I believe that the critical paradigm of Habermas (1972) (Chapter 2) and a commitment to being involved in practice and health issues wil help us to empower nursing graduates to meet future health needs of the population, and help to further needed reforms in nursing service.

POLITICAL ACTION

The assertion that nursing is therapeutic rather than simply maintaining order whilst the medical and paramedical therapists apply their interventions is threatening to a society which worships objectivity and devalues human subjectivity. The greatest challenge for the future development of therapeutic nursing is to overturn this devaluing. This can only be achieved through political means and involves educating and convincing society that the central concerns of nursing are both legitimate and important.

Confronting the notion of masculine domination

Mathews (1984) argues that women's work, and thus nursing, is devalued because it does not fit in well with the masculine view of work and suggests that:

'. . . The masculine universe must be deconstructed by an integrating feminism. By bringing together socialist feminism's structural and dynamic insights into women's material circumstances, and radical feminism's understanding of the construction of femininity and the components of consciousness, we face the possibility of an analysis of the social order and a strategy to change it that integrally incorporate women, that do not treat the masculine as universal but as a complementary part of a complex whole. The economic order is gendered and the gender order is structured economically. We can no longer work with masculine categories that prevent us from seeing this fundamental integration.'

Nurses and nursing need to confront the current domination of health care by masculinist ideology and to ensure that nursing's therapeutic potential is released.

CONCLUSION

This final chapter has attempted to overview the concept of therapeutic nursing, its evolution and its difficulties in developing its legitimacy in society. The future is truly a challenge. Challenge implies both exciting possibilities and incredible obstacles and difficulties to be overcome. Guaranteeing a future for therapeutic nursing involves both of these. Bertrand Russell said in his autobiography:

'I experienced the delight of believing that the sensible world is real. Bit by bit, chiefly under the influence of physics, this delight has faded.'

Maybe we need to be more sceptical about the view that the world is sensible and predictable, and more hopeful, assertive and confident in our ability to show others that this is so.

REFERENCES

Alfano, G.J. (1969) 'A professional approach to nursing practice', *Nursing Clinics of North America*, 4(3) 487.

Alfano, G.J. (1971) 'Healing or caretaking – which will it be?' in *Nursing Clinics of North America*, 6 273.

Ashley, J.A. (1976) *Hospitals, Paternalism, and the Role of the Nurse*, Teachers' College Press, New York.

Benner, P. (1985) *From Novice to Expert*, Addison Wesley Publishers Ltd., Menlo Park.

Bevis, E.O. (1978) *Curriculum Building in Nursing*, C.V. Mosby, St Louis.

Clay, T. (1987) *Nurses, Power and Politics*, Heineman Publishing Ltd., Oxford.

Cilliere, M.F. (1986) 'Invisible care and invisible women as health care providers',*International Journal of Nursing Studies*, **23**(2) 95–112.

Dunlop, M. (1986) 'Is a science of caring possible?' *Journal of Advanced Nursing*, **2** 661–700.

Ersser, S. (1988) 'Nursing beds and nursing therapy', in Pearson, A. (ed.) *Primary Nursing. Nursing in the Burford and Oxford Nursing Development Units*, Croom Helm, London.

Franklin, B. (1974) *Patient Anxiety on Admission to Hospital*, Royal College of Nursing Research Series, London.

Game, A. and Pringle, R. (1983) *Gender at Work*, Allen & Unwin Publishers Ltd., Sydney.

Gulino, C.K. (1983) 'Entering the mysterious dimension of other: an existential approach to nursing care', *Nursing Outlook*, **31** 352–7.

Habermann, J. (1972) *Knowledge and Human Interest* (2nd edn), Heinemanns Publishing Ltd., Oxford.

Hall, L.E. (1966) 'Another view of nursing care and quality' in Straub, M. and Parker, K. (eds), *Continuity of Patient Care: The Role of Nurses* Catholic University of America Press, Washington, DC.

McMahon, R. (1988) 'Primary nursing in practice', in Pearson, A. As above.

MacCauley, C. and Anderson, A. (1974) 'The nurse as primary therapist in the management of the patient with a stroke', *Cardiovascular Nursing*, **10** 7–10.

Marshall, S. (1987) 'The politics of prejudice', *Nursing Times*, **83**(9) 31–3.

Mason, D.J. and McCarthy, A.M. (1985) 'The politics of patient care' Mason, D.J. and Talbott, S.W. (1985) *Political Action Handbook for Nurses*, Addison Wesley, Menlo Park.

Mathews, J.J. (1984) *Good and Mad Women*, Allen & Unwin Publishers Ltd., Sydney.

Miller, A. (1985) 'A study of the dependency of elderly patients in wards using different methods of nursing care', *Age and Ageing*, **14** 132–8.

Meutzel, P.A. (1988) 'Therapeutic nursing' in Pearson, A. as above.

Nouwen, H.J.M. (1980) 'Reflections on compassion', Keynote address, Catholic Health Association of Canada.

Nuttal, P. (1983) 'Male takeover or female giveaway?', *Nursing Times*, January 12, 10–11.

Pearson, A. (1983) *The Clinical Nursing Unit*, Heinemann Publishing Ltd., Oxford.

Pearson, A. (1985) 'Introducing new norms in a nursing unit and an analysis of the process of change', unpublished PhD thesis, Department of Social Science and Administration, University of London, Goldsmiths College.

Pearson, A. (1988) *Primary Nursing – Nursing in the Burford and Oxford Nursing Development Units*, Croom Helm, London.

Pratt, A. (1980) 'Time for every purpose', Patricia Chomrley Oration, College of Nursing, Melbourne, Australia.

Reverby, S. (1987) 'A caring dilemma: womanhood and nursing an historical perspective', *Nursing Research*, **36**(1) 5–11.

Rogers, M.E. (1983) 'Beyond the horizon' in Chaska, N.L. (ed.), *The Nursing Profession: a time to speak*, McGraw-Hill, New York.

Sackett, D. *et al.* (1977) *The Role of the Nurse in Primary Health Care*, Scientific Publication **348**, The Organisation, Washington, DC.

Smuts, J.C. (1926) *Holism and Evolution*, Macmillan, New York.

Tiffany, D.H. (1977) 'Nursing organisational structure and the real goals of hospitals', unpublished PhD thesis, Indiana University.

Vance, C.N., Talbott, S.W., McBride, A.B. and Mason, D.J. (1985) 'Coming of age: the women's movement and nursing', in Mason, D.J. and Talbott, S.W. (eds) *Political Action Handbook for Nurses*, Addison-Wesley, Menlo Park.

Weinberg, R., Lilijestrand, J. and Moroe, S. (1983) 'Inpatient management by a nurse practitioner: effectiveness in a rehabilitation setting', *Archives of Physical Medicine and Rehabilitation*, **64** 588–90.

Index